GIVING CARDIOVASCULAR DRUGS SAFELY

GIVING CARDIOVASCULAR DRUGS SAFELY

Nursing78 Books
Intermed Communications, Inc.
Horsham, Pennsylvania

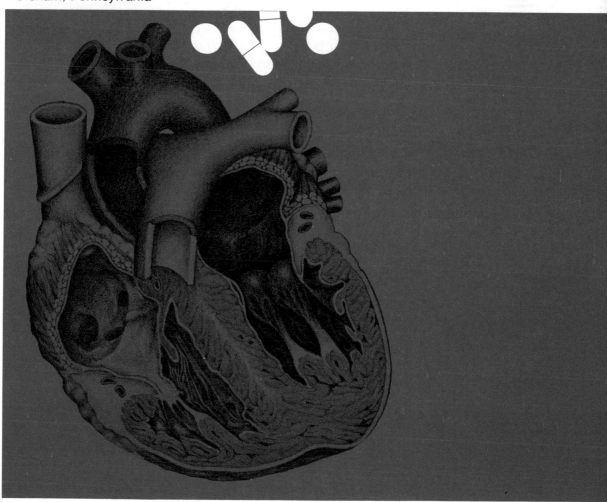

NURSING78 BOOKS

PUBLISHER: Eugene W. Jackson
Editorial Director: Daniel L. Cheney
Clinical Director: Margaret Van Meter, RN
Graphics Director: John Isely
Business Manager: Tom Temple

NURSING78 SKILLBOOK SERIES
Editorial staff for this volume:
Book Editor: Jean Robinson
Clinical Editors: Barbara McVan, RN, Virginia Jackle, RN, and
 Minnie Rose, RN, BSN, MEd
Marginalia Editor: Avery Rome
Assistant Editors: Vonda Heller, and Karen Kotz, RN
Copy Editors: Patricia A. Hamilton, Kathy Lorenc
Production Manager: Bernard Haas
Production Assistants: David C. Kosten, Margie Tyson
Designer: Maggie Arnott
Artists: Elizabeth Clark, Owen Heinrich, Kim Milnazic, Robert Renn,
 Sandra Simms, and James Storey

Clinical consultants

Michael R. Cohen, BS Pharm., *Assistant Director of Pharmacy (Clinical Services)
Temple University Hospital, Philadelphia, Pa.*

Catherine Ciaverelli Manzi, RN, *Head Nurse, Coronary Care Unit, Hospital of
Philadelphia College of Osteopathic Medicine, Philadelphia, Pa.*

Peter G. Lavine, MD, *Director of Coronary Care Unit, Crozer-Chester Medical
Center, Chester, Pa.*

Library of Congress catalog card number 77-20635 ISBN 0-916730-07-7

CONTENTS

Guide to drug charts
The symbol ◇ after a trade name indicates that the drug is also available in Canada.
The symbol ◇◇ means that the drug is available in Canda only.
Unmarked trade names mean that the drug is available only in the United States.
The symbol G stands for gram.
These symbols will be used in all the drug charts throughout the book.

PATIENT TEACHING AIDS

AUTHORS

Michael R. Cohen is the assistant director of pharmacy (clinical services) at the Temple University Hospital, Philadelphia, Pa., as well as an instructor in clinical pharmacy at the Temple School of Pharmacy. Mr. Cohen was one of the advisors on this book. He received his BS in pharmacy at Temple University, Philadelphia.

John A. Gans is an associate professor of clinical pharmacy at the Philadelphia College of Pharmacy and Science, Philadelphia, Pa. He received his PharmD from the Philadelphia College of Pharmacy.

Edmund J. Haughey, Jr. is the assistant director of pharmacy services at the Presbyterian Hospital, University of Pennsylvania Medical Center, Philadelphia, Pa. He is also an instructor in clinical pharmacy at the Philadelphia College of Pharmacy and Science, where he received his PharmD.

Daniel A. Hussar is dean of faculty and Remington Professor at the Philadelphia College of Pharmacy and Science, Philadelphia. He received his BS, MS, and PhD from the Philadelphia College of Pharmacy and Science.

Catherine Ciaverelli Manzi is the head nurse of the coronary care unit, Hospital of the Philadelphia College of Osteopathic Medicine, Philadelphia, Pa. She is a graduate of the Hahnemann Hospital School of Nursing, Philadelphia, and a member of the American Association of Critical Care Nurses. Ms. Manzi was one of the advisors on this book.

Frances M. Sica is a clinical pharmacist at the Presbyterian Hospital, University of Pennsylvania Medical Center, Philadelphia, Pa. She received her BS from the Philadelphia College of Pharmacy and Science.

Paula Brammer Vetter is a staff development instructor of the coronary care unit, Cleveland Clinic Hospital, Cleveland, Ohio. She received her BSN from the College of Mount Saint Joseph-on-the-Ohio, Cincinnati, Ohio. Ms. Vetter is a certified CPR instructor with the American Heart Association and a member of the American Association of Critical Care Nurses.

Gayle Whitman is assistant head nurse of the cardiovascular intensive care unit at the Cleveland Clinic Hospital, Cleveland, Ohio. She received her BSN from the University of Pittsburgh, and is presently working on her MSN at Case Western Reserve University. Ms. Whitman is a member of the American Association of Critical Care Nurses.

Frank F. Williams is the drug information pharmacist at Temple University Hospital, Philadelphia, Pa., as well as adjunct assistant clinical professor at the Temple University School of Pharmacy. He received his PharmD from the Philadelphia College of Pharmacy and Science.

FOREWORD

Why a book just about cardiovascular drugs, you may ask. Well, keeping current about all drugs is an ongoing challenge for all nurses. And surely, cardiovascular drugs are among the most paradoxical. Given correctly, these drugs can *save* lives. But given incorrectly — or unwisely — they can *take* lives. And many times, the nurse's knowledge is what determines the outcome.

But, are you involved with cardiovascular drugs? Probably you are, whether you realize it now or not. Because, according to the latest statistics from the American Heart Association, well over 29 million Americans have some form of heart or blood vessel disease. Moreover, cardiovascular disease will be responsible for approximately 52% of all deaths this year. These figures attest to the problem's magnitude, and justify the millions of dollars spent annually on research for prevention or treatment.

That's one of the reasons this book is so valuable. It'll help you see how cardiovascular disease — and the drugs used to treat it — affect all nursing fields. Patients taking these drugs are everywhere — in the doctor's office, as well as on every floor of the hospital. Situations in which you must administer the drugs, or simply know how they work, are endless. A patient's life can literally depend on what you remember.

GIVING CARDIOVASCULAR DRUGS SAFELY will *help* you remember. Unlike many other nursing books, which have a preponderance of pharmacology, this Skillbook presents the major classes of drugs in language easy to understand. Most important, it tells you what you, as a *nurse,* should know about the drugs — so you can help the patient.

Besides the text, this Skillbook contains many handy reference guides: a dosage and side effects chart for each major class of drugs and — in most chapters — drug interaction charts. You'll also find onset-of-action graphs, pertinent EKG strips, blood data about drug toxicities, and a handy dosage calculator. Near the beginning of the book is a well-designed chart that will help you review drug actions on the autonomic nervous system. At the back of this Skillbook is a helpful glossary.

One of the finest — and most unique — features of this Skillbook, however, is its emphasis on patient teaching. What to tell the patient about his therapy is discussed thoroughly in every chapter, of course. But additional teaching tools are added: easy-to-understand patient teaching cards for commonly prescribed drugs, and helpful diets and food charts that may be needed to accompany the drugs. *All of these may be reproduced on your office or hospital copier and given to patients.*

As I conclude my introduction to this unusual book on cardiovascular drugs, an old saying comes to mind: "When opportunity knocks, open the door." Before you is an opportunity — an opportunity to learn about current drug therapy for cardiovascular disease, to enhance patient care, and to develop self-confidence and professional pride. Make the most of it!

—EDITH McCARTER, RN, CVS, MS
Director
Cardiovascular Nurse Specialist Program
Arizona Heart Institute
Phoenix, Arizona

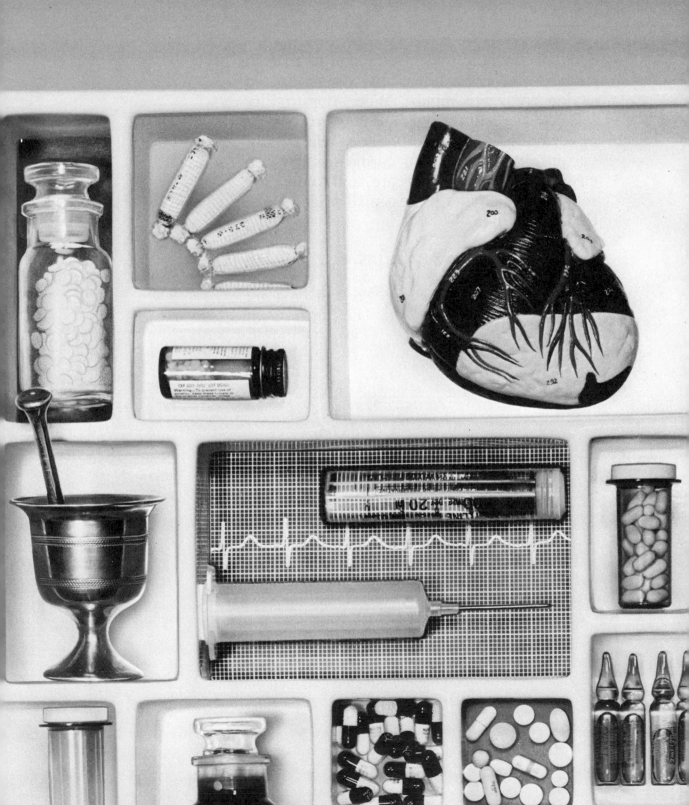

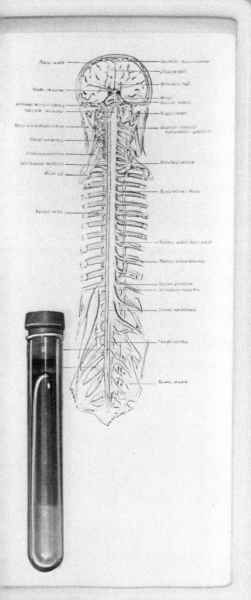
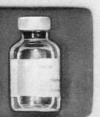
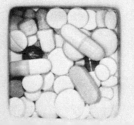

BEGIN WITH BASICS

Here's a brief,
but comprehensive,
review of the
cardiovascular
system
and the ANS.

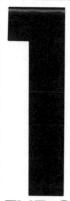

THE CARDIOVASCULAR SYSTEM AND THE A.N.S.: Reviewing the basics

BY PAULA BRAMMER VETTER, RN, BSN

TO UNDERSTAND HOW cardiovascular drugs work, you need to know the cardiovascular system's workings — its anatomy and physiology. Dull stuff? Complicated? Yes, a little, but it's also fascinating.

Here's a brief description you really ought to review — even though you may have covered it in school. It'll help you better understand how certain drugs act on the cardiovascular system.

The body's pump

The heart is an impeccably designed muscular pump connected to a "superhighway" transport system of blood vessels which traverse the entire body. Not only does this system circulate oxygen and nutrient-rich blood throughout the body, it also rids the body of waste materials.

The heart is enclosed in a fibrous, protective sac — the pericardium. If you were to open the pericardium, you'd see the shiny red membranous surface of the heart; this surface is the epicardium. It covers the heart muscle and supports it. Strip away the epicardium, and you'd see the myocardium; this is the heart muscle that does the pumping. On the heart's interior surface, lining the chambers and covering valves and associated structures, lies a shiny, endothelial membrane called the endocardium. The endocardium provides a smooth, non-traumatic surface for the blood to pass over as it circulates through the heart. If the endocardium becomes scarred or rough, it can break down fragile blood platelets passing over it and increase the chance of clotting.

In normal adults, the heart is approximately 5 inches long, about 3½ inches in diameter at its widest point, and weighs between 250 and 300 grams. It's located substernally just about in the mid-line with its apex pointing left. The heart, which is divided into four chambers (two atria and two ventricles), is also rotated slightly so that the right ventricle lies in front of the left ventricle. From the front, you regard the right ventricle as the anterior ventricle and the left ventricle as the posterior.

The thin-walled atria serve as reservoirs and booster pumps to increase blood volume in the ventricles, which fill primarily by gravity. Blood rushes into the ventricles from the atria when the valves between them open: the tricuspid valve separating the right atrium from the right ventricle, and the mitral valve separating the left atrium. Then, a fraction of a second before the ventricles contract, the atria squeeze still more blood — another 20% — into the ventricles' chambers. This "atrial kick," as it is called, contributes significantly to the stroke volume (the amount of blood ejected from the ventricles with each systole).

The heart: two pumps in one
To understand the heart's function, divide it into two segments:
- a low-pressure pump (right atrium and ventricle)
- a high-pressure pump (left atrium and ventricle)

Here's how the right-sided, low-pressure pump supplies the pulmonary vasculature. The right atrium receives venous blood from the systemic circulation via the superior and inferior vena cavae. This deoxygenated blood then flows across the tricuspid valve into the right ventricle.

There, it gets ejected with ventricular systole through the pulmonary outflow tract and into the pulmonary artery. Because the pulmonary arterial system is a *low-pressure* system with a mean pressure of approximately 15mm of mercury, it doesn't require much energy to propel blood into the pulmonary circuit and overcome the slight resistance of the pulmonary vasculature. Thus, the right ventricle can function almost as simply as a fireplace bellows. Its crescent-shaped interior squeezes together in ventricular systole, opening the pulmonic valve and ejecting 70 to 80 cc of blood into the pulmonary artery.

From the pulmonary artery, the blood enters the pulmonary capillary bed where gas exchange takes place. Freshly oxygenated blood then flows through four pulmonary veins into the posterior portion of the left atrium. The mitral valve opens, releasing blood into the left ventricle, and finally the ventricle contracts, propelling blood into the systemic arterial circulation.

The left ventricle is about three times as thick as the right ventricle, and unlike the right ventricle, is a *high* pressure pump. Why is this so? Well, each left ventricular systole pumps against a mean systemic arterial pressure of 90 to 120 mm Hg, which is greater than pulmonary circuit pressure. To eject adequate volume against this pressure, the left ventricle has a specialized structure — a cone-shaped cavity surrounded by multiple muscle layers arranged longitudinally, horizontally, and diagonally. Ventricular systole occurs when a "wringing" motion propels blood forcefully enough to overcome systemic vascular resistance. You could call the left ventricle's muscle wall the real powerhouse of the heart. Ninety-five percent of the energy expended by the heart goes to open the aortic valve and initiate systole.

Depolarization and repolarization

Now that we've reviewed the mechanics of systole and myocardial contraction, let's look at the physiological processes that start things happening. First, imagine a single myocardial cell — of protein filaments of actin and myosin — suspended in a gelatinous substance called sarcoplasm. The fluid within and outside the cell differs: Intracellular fluid is rich in potassium while extracellular fluid contains more sodium.

When electrical current, generated by the heart's pacemaker, reaches the cell, it creates an ionic imbalance. Potassium moves out of the cell while sodium migrates inward (depolarization). Calcium, which was previously bound to

Take heart

An astounding piece of machinery, the healthy adult heart weighs approximately 11 ounces and beats 100,000 times a day (2.5 billion times in a lifetime). It circulates eight pints of blood continuously, in a day, pumping the equivalent of 4,300 gallons of oxygen-rich blood along 60,000 miles of blood vessels to nourish the body.

With computer-like efficiency, the cardiovascular system can increase the flow of blood to areas that need it. During exertion, as you know, the heart's output increases: The pulse rate goes up, you breathe faster, and the blood vessels dilate so that the body's organs and tissues can extract more oxygen from the bloodstream.

When the heart doesn't work efficiently, the patient's life is threatened. More Americans and Canadians die from heart disease than from all other causes combined. (Heart disease kills one million Americans annually.) The more you know about the heart's action and the cardiovascular system, the better care you can give to cardiac patients.

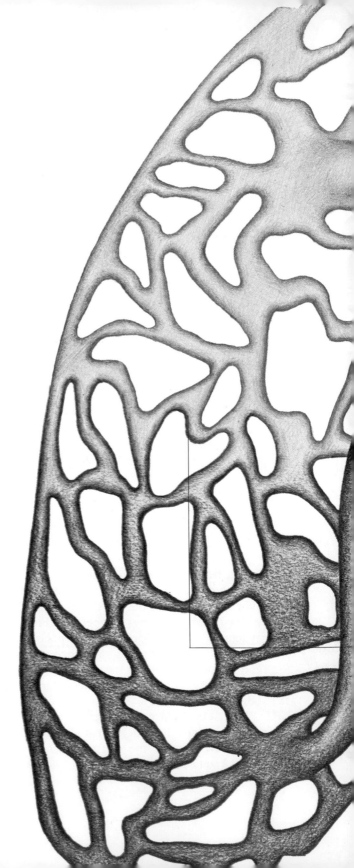

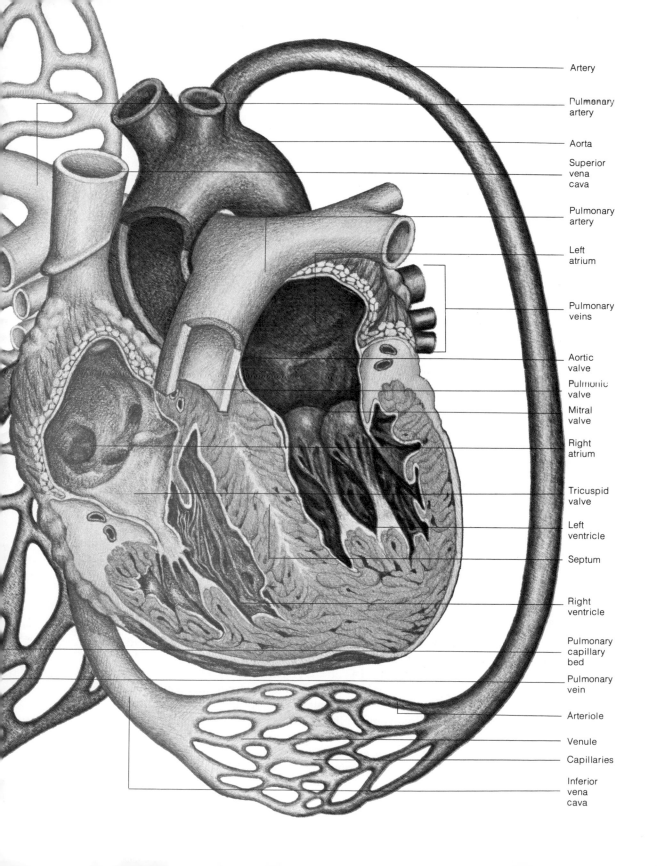

Artery

Pulmonary
artery

Aorta

Superior
vena
cava

Pulmonary
artery

Left
atrium

Pulmonary
veins

Aortic
valve

Pulmonic
valve

Mitral
valve

Right
atrium

Tricuspid
valve

Left
ventricle

Septum

Right
ventricle

Pulmonary
capillary
bed

Pulmonary
vein

Arteriole

Venule

Capillaries

Inferior
vena
cava

structures within the cell, is liberated and makes actin and myosin filaments slide across one another. This causes cell shortening and muscle contraction. After contraction, though, the calcium is reabsorbed almost immediately, allowing the cell to repolarize (repolarization). The sodium and potassium return to their original positions, as do the actin and myosin filaments. Now, the cell is ready to respond to another stimulus.

Later on in this book, you'll learn how inotropic drugs are used to control heart muscle contractions. Inotropic drugs affect the *force* with which the heart contracts, thereby affecting its output. For example, a positive inotropic drug (digitalis) increases contractility, whereas a negative inotropic agent (propranolol) decreases contractility.

What the pacemaker does

The electrical energy causing depolarization is generated and discharged at regular intervals by special pacemaker cells within the myocardium. These pacemaker cells are connected by glycogen-rich conduction pathways which carry the electrical current to all parts of the myocardium. Of course, this current can move through the myocardium without these pathways, but their presence makes conduction more efficient. Current travels approximately seven times as fast through the conduction pathways as it does through the general myocardial tissue.

The heart's normal pacemaker is the sinoatrial (SA) node, a body of specialized pacemaker tissue located high in the right atrium near the inflow tract of the superior and inferior vena cava. In most adults, the node discharges electrical energy at a rhythmic rate of 60 to 100 impulses per minute. The conduction pathways carry these impulses through the atrial tissue and down to the atrioventricular (AV) node located near the intraventricular septum just adjacent to the tricuspid valve. Impulses are delayed for several milliseconds in the AV node, to prevent the ventricles from being stimulated at inordinately rapid rates by the atria, and to permit adequate time for the ventricle to fill adequately before its systole.

Connected to the AV node is a thick bundle of conducting nerve fibers known as the bundle of His. These fibers divide to form a left and a right bundle branch; then the left branch divides once again into anterior and posterior branches. These

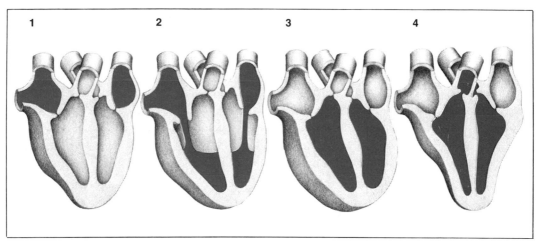

three bundle branches carry current through the ventricles to the end of the conduction system, or the Purkinje fibers. The microscopic Purkinje fibers emerge from the bundle branches and are imbedded in the myocardium; they transfer impulses to the ventricular muscle, causing depolarization and contraction.

If the SA node fails, the heart has a protective back-up system of auxillary pacemakers which continue to stimulate the myocardium: For example, the AV node can do this if necessary. However, the AV node discharges electrical stimuli at a slower rate (40 to 60 times per minute) than the SA node. This keeps the two pacemakers from competing with each other during normal SA node functioning.

If the SA node and AV node both fail, the ventricular muscle fibers continue to depolarize by themselves. This is called inherent rhythmicity. The ventricular muscle fibers' rate is even slower (approximately 20-40 times per minute); and though it provides minimal perfusion of vital organs, it usually produces serious symptoms.

How cardiovascular drugs affect EKGs
You can see the depolarization-repolarization process in electrocardiograms. You can learn more about interpreting them in the Nursing Skillbook READING EKGs CORRECTLY. In this book, you'll learn how drugs affect the *normal* EKG.

The normal EKG has three main components: The P wave shows atrial depolarization; the QRS complex shows ventricu-

Changes of heart
The drawings above show the changes the heart goes through during a single cardiac cycle:
1. Used blood from the body enters the right atrium at the same time that oxygenated blood from the lungs enters the left atrium;
2. An impulse from the sinoatrial node causes both atria to contract, pushing blood through the mitral and tricuspid valves into the ventricles;
3. Blood remains in the ventricles for milliseconds (the only time the heart is still) until an impulse from the atrioventricular node triggers a contraction;
4. Both ventricles contract, pushing stale blood to the lungs and fresh blood to the body.

THE BASIC EKG COMPLEX: A REVIEW

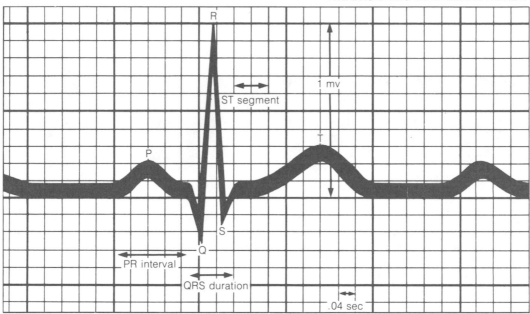

lar depolarization; and the T wave shows that the ventricles have repolarized and are ready for another stimulus. (Atrial repolarization is seldom seen because it occurs simultaneously with the QRS and is masked by this dominant complex.) The interval from the beginning of the P wave to the beginning of the QRS shows how long the impulse takes to travel from the atria to the ventricular muscle fibers. If this interval is too long, there's an atrioventricular conduction problem.

The duration of the QRS complex measures the time needed to activate ventricular muscle mass. Prolongation of this interval means a conduction problem within the ventricles.

Drugs affect the EKG by acting on various parts of the heart. For example, digitalis slows conduction through the upper and lower portions of the AV node; propranolol slows conduction through its center. Thus, a patient who receives both drugs simultaneously may have a prolonged P-R interval that is a drug-induced heart block. You'll learn how other drugs can affect a patient's EKG in other chapters.

Arteries, capillaries, and veins
Now that we've discussed the heart's work as a pump, let's

look at the vessels connected to the pump. In the high-pressure arterial system, large arteries branch into smaller arteries, and finally into arterioles. The arterioles regulate most blood flow; their strong muscular walls can decrease a vessel's diameter to one-fourth of its former size after a cue from the autonomic nervous system, or from local autoregulation which we'll discuss shortly.

Because they can constrict and redirect blood flow, the arterioles can compensate for a 15% to 25% blood volume deficit before there's a significant change in systolic blood pressure. The arterioles also respond to vasodilating drugs; a sufficient dose can increase their capacity by 1.5 to 2 liters, improving blood flow, whereas a vasoconstrictor can decrease their capacity by 1 to 1.5 liters, restricting blood flow.

The arterioles eventually branch into capillary networks. There, diffusion takes place between the blood and interstitial fluid. The capillaries then form venules and finally veins. These are the reservoir for circulating blood, and contain about half the body's supply. The pulmonary venous system also contains a significant volume of blood; in fact, vessels within the lungs can withstand a three-fold increase in blood flow before the pulmonary arterial pressure rises appreciably.

Large veins offer considerable resistance to blood flow, whereas resistance encountered in the smaller veins is significantly less. Unidirectional valves in the large veins plus leg muscle contraction propel blood back toward the heart against gravity. This reduces pressure within the dependent veins.

The heart's blood supply

Three major coronary arteries nourish the myocardium: the right coronary, the left anterior descending, and the circumflex artery. The left anterior and circumflex artery arise from a common artery called the left main trunk. These arteries originate in the aorta at the cusps of the aortic valve. How well they work depends on three things: systemic blood pressure, heart rate and rhythm, and circulatory load.

In most people, the right coronary artery supplies blood to the SA and the AV nodes and the right ventricular wall — right coronary dominance. It also supplies the bundle of His and the inferior (diaphragmatic) wall of the left ventricle. (In some people the left coronary artery is dominant.)

The left anterior descending coronary artery supplies the

HOW THE AUTONOMIC NERVOUS SYSTEM WORKS

What regulates the cardiovascular system? The autonomic nervous system (ANS), and to some degree, local autoregulatory mechanisms. The ANS regulates body functions we can't control by will; for example, blood pressure, water balance, and digestion.

It has two divisions: sympathetic and parasympathetic. The sympathetic system regulates the body's expenditure of energy, especially in times of stress. The parasympathetic system regulates the body's "domestic" functions and helps it conserve energy. Both receive their orders from the central nervous system.

Let's see how this works. The figure at right shows how nerve cell bodies for the sympathetic system are located in the part of the spinal cord that runs through the chest and lumbar region of the back. When impulses from the CNS reach these bodies, they travel along preganglionic nerve fibers to a second relay station outside the spinal column called a ganglion. From the ganglion, they proceed to their destination (heart, bladder, liver, stomach,

eye). Here they trigger the release of a catecholamine, norepinephrine. These nerves are adrenergic.

Nerve cell bodies for the parasympathetic system are located in the extreme ends of the spinal cord. Like the sympathetic system, they transmit impulses from the CNS along preganglionic nerve fibers, but their second relay stations (ganglia) are located in the organ involved. Here they trigger the release of the neurohormone acetylcholine. These nerves are called cholinergic.

The sympathetic division of the autonomic nervous system has two types of receptor cells that respond to stimulation: alpha and beta (B1 and B2) receptors.

In the figure below, you can see what happens to various parts of the body when norepinephrine or acetylcholine are released. Biochemical changes take place within the cells causing smooth muscle to contract or relax. These effects can be mimicked or blocked by certain drugs.

For example, overstimulation of the parasympathetic system will

decrease heart rate, leading to bradycardia. The anticholinergic drug atropine, which blocks the body's response to acetylcholine, turns this response around. It increases the heart rate, so the drug is useful as an antiarrhythmic.

The way body organs or structures respond to stimulation in the sympathetic division depends on the type of receptor. For example, cutaneous blood vessels have alpha receptors. They respond to the release of norepinephrine by constricting. This response can be blocked with an alpha receptor blocker such as phentolamine.

Beta responses can be blocked by propranolol. The figure below shows how it slows down the heart, which is why it's an antiarrhythmic. However, when a patient also has asthma, propranolol is contraindicated: It blocks bronchiole response, causing constriction.

You'll read how other drugs mimic or block the effects of the catecholamines further along in this book. Use this section to help you to understand them better.

HOW DRUGS BLOCK AUTONOMIC NERVOUS SYSTEM RESPONSES

PARASYMPATHETIC		INNERVATED ORGAN	SYMPATHETIC		
			ALPHA	BETA 1	BETA 2
▼	▲	Heart		▲▽	
▲	▼	Bronchioles			▼▲
▲	▼	GI Tract			
▲	▼	Bladder			
▼	▲	Bladder sphincter			
▼	▲	Blood vessels	▲▼*		▼▲**
▲	▼	Sweat and salivary glands			

▲ ▼ Major parasympathetic response triggered by body's natural release of the neurohormone acetylcholine (ACH). These nerve fibers are called cholinergic

▲ ▼ Here's what happens when atropine and other drugs with anticholinergic effects are given

△ ▽ Major sympathetic (adrenergic) response triggered by body's natural release of epinephrine and norepinephrine

▲ ▼ Here's what happens when antiadrenergic drugs dibenzyline, phentolamine, and tolazoline are given

▲ ▼ Here's what happens when antiadrenergic drug, propranolol, is given

▲ Constricts or stimulates   ▼ Relaxes or dilates   ** Skeletal muscle   * Cutaneous

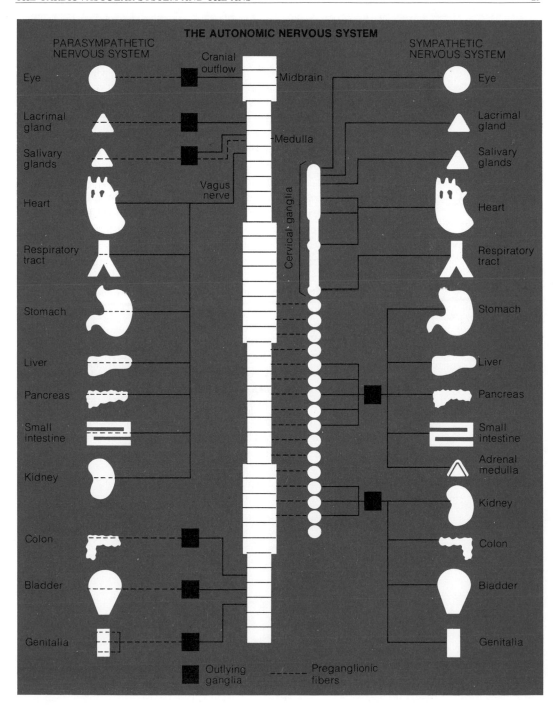

THE AUTONOMIC NERVOUS SYSTEM

PARASYMPATHETIC NERVOUS SYSTEM

SYMPATHETIC NERVOUS SYSTEM

Eye

Lacrimal gland

Salivary glands

Heart

Respiratory tract

Stomach

Liver

Pancreas

Small intestine

Kidney

Colon

Bladder

Genitalia

Cranial outflow

Midbrain

Medulla

Vagus nerve

Cervical ganglia

Eye

Lacrimal gland

Salivary glands

Heart

Respiratory tract

Stomach

Liver

Pancreas

Small intestine

Adrenal medulla

Kidney

Colon

Bladder

Genitalia

Outlying ganglia

Preganglionic fibers

bundle branches and the anterior wall of the left ventricle. The circumflex artery delivers blood to the lateral and posterior walls of the left ventricle. The coronary veins follow the same route as the arteries; they return blood to the right atrium for transport to the lungs for oxygenation.

The coronary arteries fill up primarily during diastole, or the resting phase of the heart. If you have a patient with a rapid heart rate, he has a two-fold problem. His rapid rate means that the period of diastole is shortened. His heart not only works harder than before and requires more oxygen to meet its needs, it also gets less oxygen than it did at normal rates. Because of this, the patient has chest pain. Once his tachycardia is alleviated, his pain may subside without further treatment. His heart was only demanding adequate time for proper coronary artery perfusion.

Good coronary perfusion also takes adequate systemic arterial pressure. When below 60 mm Hg, the low pressure will almost always hamper coronary circulation.

Achieving optimal performance
How well the cardiovascular system operates depends on these things: the heart's filling pressure during diastole; the resistance against which it pumps; its contractile force; its rate, its conduction system; the synchronized mechanical contraction of atria and ventricles; and the body's metabolism. As we have explained, this system can compensate for many defects that arise. However, when it fails to do so, we can intervene with the best cardiovascular drugs.

SKILLCHECK 1

1. A normal adult's heart is about 5" long, 3½" in diameter at its widest point, and weighs about _____.
   a) 10-20 G
   b) 250-300 G
   c) 500-600 G

2. The interior surface of the heart, which is composed of endothelial membrane, is called the _____.
   a) myocardium
   b) pericardium
   c) endocardium

3. The right atrium of the heart is separated from the right ventricle by the _____ valve.
   a) tricuspid
   b) mitral
   c) pulmonic

4. When an ionic imbalance is created in the heart's cells, depolarization occurs and _____ moves out of cells.
   a) potassium
   b) sodium
   c) calcium

5. During depolarization, _____ migrates into cells.
   a) calcium
   b) potassium
   c) sodium

6. The conduction pathways of the myocardium carry electrical impulses _____ times as fast as general myocardial tissue.
   a) 30
   b) 7
   c) 12

7. Impulses are delayed several milliseconds in the _____ to prevent the ventricles from being too rapidly stimulated by the atria.
   a) AV node
   b) SA node
   c) outlying ganglia

8. The AV node discharges electrical stimuli at a rate of _____ per minute.
   a) 60-80
   b) 40-60
   c) 20-40

9. A sufficient dose of vasodilator can increase the arterioles' capacity by about _____ liters.
   a) ¼-½
   b) 3-4
   c) 1½-2

10. The major coronary arteries are the right coronary, the left anterior descending, and the _____.
    a) the pulmonary artery
    b) the left circumflex artery
    c) the right anterior descending artery

11. In most people, blood is supplied to the SA and AV nodes and the right ventricle by the _____ artery.
    a) right coronary
    b) left anterior descending
    c) pulmonary

12. Sympathetic nervous system receptor cells that respond to the body's natural release of epinephrine and norepinephrine are called _____.
    a) adrenergic
    b) cholinergic
    c) inotropic

13. Parasympathetic nervous system fibers trigger the release of acetylcholine and are called _____.
    a) adrenergic
    b) cholinergic
    c) autoregulatory

14. Overstimulation of the parasympathetic nervous system will _____ heart rate.
    a) increase
    b) decrease
    c) both of these

15. Cutaneous blood vessels, which have alpha receptors, respond to the release of norepinephrine by _____.
    a) dilating
    b) constricting
    c) distending

16. Propranolol can slow down the heart rate because it blocks the responses of _____ receptors.
    a) alpha
    b) beta
    c) parasympathetic

(Answers on page 165)

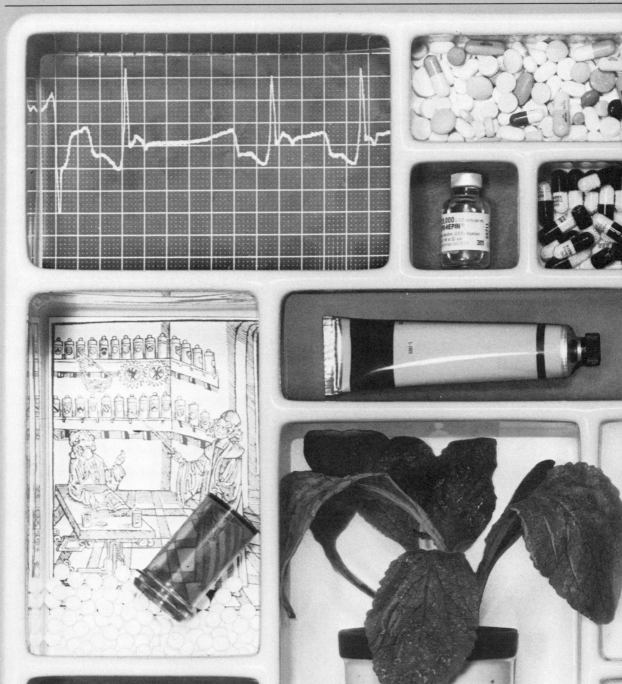

CARDIAC THERAPY

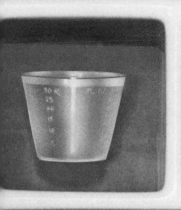

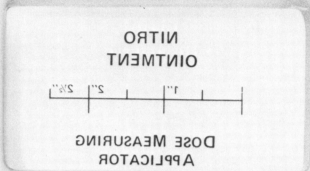

NITRO
OINTMENT

| 2¼" | 2" | 1" | |

DOSE MEASURING
APPLICATOR

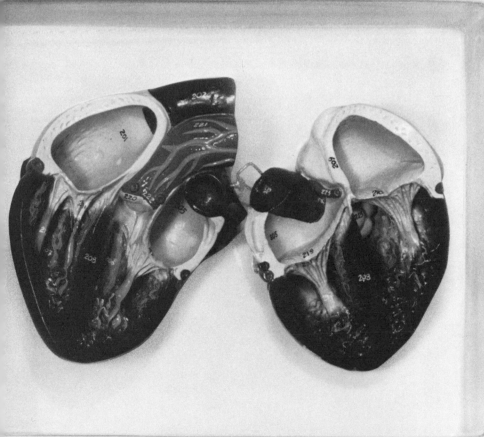

The facts about the basic drugs you'll be working with — digitalis glycosides… diuretics… vasodilators, and anti-arrhythmics.

2

DIGITALIS GLYCOSIDES: Keeping them therapeutic, not toxic

BY JOHN A. GANS, PharmD

NOT LONG AGO, 68-year-old Mr. Haines, a diabetic, entered the emergency room of a large Philadelphia hospital. He complained of dyspnea and orthopnea and showed signs of congestive heart failure. He was digitalized over the next 5 days with intravenous and oral digoxin and then placed on a maintenance dosage of 0.25 mg of digoxin daily. On the 9th day, he recovered sufficiently to be discharged under the care of his family doctor. He returned home with prescriptions for digoxin, hydrochlorothiazide, potassium chloride syrup, and tolbutamide.

Mr. Haines, unfortunately, was no expert in self-administration of such a complex drug regimen. And like so many patients on digitalis therapy, he received little instruction about his drugs before he left the hospital. What happened to Mr. Haines three months later might have been prevented if he'd understood the purpose of his drug therapy, the necessity for continued medical supervision, and the importance of taking the drugs as prescribed. Someone should have told Mr. Haines which symptoms suggest digitalis toxicity and told him to call his doctor if any of them occurred.

You'll find out what happened to Mr. Haines later in this

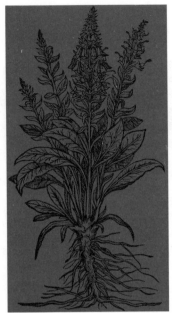

A plant for all seasons
Since the time of the ancient
Egyptians, plants containing
cardiac glycosides have been
used as medicine. And doctors,
over the ages, have prescribed
foxglove, or digitalis for ailments
ranging from epilepsy to skin
ulcers.

The first scientific treatise on
the subject was published in 1785
by William Withering. In it, he
outlined the use of digitalis for
dropsy but made only a passing
reference to its effect on the heart.
Unfortunately, the guidelines he
suggested for the plant's safe use
went largely unheeded. For over a
century, people continued to use
digitalis, often in toxic doses, for
any number of disorders.

Finally, digitalis came into its
own as a cardiac drug in the 20th
century. Doctors prescribed it
mostly for atrial fibrillation at first.
But within the past 60 years,
they've recognized its main value
— to treat congestive heart failure.

chapter. He's a classic example of what can go wrong for one
of your patients taking digitalis glycosides if you and he aren't
informed. Inadequate instruction for prolonged self-
medication is always a serious matter, but especially so when
one of the digitalis glycosides is involved. These indispensible
agents for managing congestive heart failure and certain arrhythmias are among the most complex to manage successfully.

Your role in digitalis therapy
Although digitalis has been used for 200 years to treat cardiac
disease, there are still no standardized procedures for its administration. The range between therapeutic and toxic effects
is narrow and may be adversely affected by concurrent disease, drug interaction, or the patient's age. Even a prescribed
maintenance dosage of digitalis may later become toxic for a
variety of reasons.

Because we lack standardized regimens, patient care places
great demands upon the skill and experience of those administering digitalis glycosides. As a nurse, you must:
• Recognize signs of toxicity.
• Help prevent drug interactions.
• Take a leading role in teaching hospitalized and ambulatory patients self-administraton and safe use of these and other
drugs.

What digitalis glycosides do
No one knows exactly how digitalis glycosides work, but the
mechanism of action and the therapeutic effects of the various
forms are essentially the same. However, they differ significantly in how they're administered, how fast they're absorbed
and excreted by the body, and how long they act.

They help the failing or arrhythmic heart by:
1. Increasing the force of myocardial contractions and improving cardiac efficiency.
2. Lengthening the refractory period and reducing the heart
rate by slowing the rate of impulse transmission in the conduction tissues.

Digitalis relieves congestive heart failure directly. The heart
muscle contracts more forcefully and at a slower rate — per-
mitting it to fill and empty more blood from its chambers with
each beat. This improves the patient's pulmonary and sys-

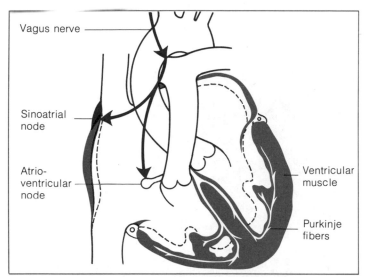

Vagus nerve

Sinoatrial node

Atrio-ventricular node

Ventricular muscle

Purkinje fibers

Faint heart never won
Digitalis helps to strengthen the failing heart, increasing its output as much as 30%. Although doctors don't yet know how digitalis works, this is what it does:
● increases the vagal tone, which slows the heart's action;
● slows the conduction through the AV node, which allows more time for blood to enter the ventricles;
● increases the force of ventricular contractions, which sends more blood to the lungs and the body.

temic circulation, and with it the overall performance of body organs. The increased cardiac output improves flow to kidneys and increases urine formation. Venous pressure falls, enabling edema in the lungs, abdomen, legs, and other areas to be diminished or completely abolished through improved kidney function. Heart size decreases (in many cases to normal) through the enriching effects of restored blood flow.

The effect of digitalis on conduction tissue also controls atrial arrhythmias (atrial flutter, atrial fibrillation, paroxysmal tachycardia). It slows the transmission of impulses from the atria, thereby protecting the ventricles from overstimulation. By doing so, it reduces the number of ineffective beats and restores the heart to a more normal rate.

Many doctors prefer oral administration of digitalis glycosides because that's safest and most economical. In most cases, they don't order intramuscular and subcutaneous injections because of the drugs' locally irritating effects and uncertain absorption. When digitalis glycosides must be given parenterally, the doctor usually chooses the intravenous route. He selects this route when rapid digitalization is indicated, as in severe pulmonary edema caused by acute left-sided heart failure, and when oral administration is impossible, as in coma or vomiting.

But oral administration has its drawback. The rate of the drugs' absorption by the body is somewhat unpredictable.

NURSES' GUIDE TO
DIGITALIS GLYCOSIDES

GENERIC NAME	TRADE NAME	ROUTE AND DOSAGE	TOXIC EFFECTS
digitoxin	Digitoxin◇ Purodigin◇ Crystodigin	P.O.: Digitalization 1.2-2.0 mg. Initial dose 0.6 mg, followed by 0.4 mg, then 0.2 mg q4-6h. Slow digitalization dose 0.2 mg b.i.d. for 4 days. Maintenance 0.05-0.3 mg daily. I.V.: Digitalization 1.2-1.6 mg. Initial dose 0.6 mg, followed by 0.4 mg 4-6h later, then 0.2 mg q4-6h until therapeutic effect apparent (should occur in 8-12h). Maintenance 0.05-0.3 mg daily I.V. or P.O.	Anorexia, nausea, vomiting, diarrhea, abdominal discomfort, headache, fatigue, restlessness, irritability, confusion and disorientation (especially in elderly), blurred or yellow vision, flickering lights, white borders around dark objects, colored dots, excessive slowing of pulse, all arrhythmias, especially PVCs in adults
digitalis	Digitalis◇ Digifortis Pil-Digis	P.O.: Digitalization total dose 1-2 G in equal parts given q6h. Maintenance 50-400 mg daily.	
lanatoside C	Cedilanid◇	P.O.: Digitalization 5-10 mg in daily decreasing doses. First day-3.5 mg, second day-2.5 mg, third day-2 mg, then 1.5 mg daily until full digitalization obtained. Maintenance 0.5-1.5 mg daily.	
deslanoside (desacetyl-lanatoside C)	Cedilanid-D	I.V., I.M.: Digitalization 1.6 mg I.M. in 2 doses over 12h, 1.6 mg I.V. in 1 or 2 doses over 12h. For maintenance, start lanatoside C within 12 hours.	
digoxin	Digoxin Lanoxin◇ Novodigoxin◇◇ Rougoxin◇◇	P.O.: Digitalization 1.0-1.5 mg. Initial dose 0.5-0.75 mg, then 0.25-0.5 mg q6-8h until therapeutic effect attained. Maintenance 0.125-0.5 mg daily (0.125-0.25 mg in elderly patients) I.V., I.M.: Digitalization 0.5-1.5 mg. Initial dose 0.25-0.5 mg, then 0.25 mg q4-6h. Maintenance 0.125-0.5 mg daily (average 0.25 mg)	
ouabain (G-strophanthin)	Ouabain	I.V.: 0.5-1.0 mg, initial dose 0.25-0.50 mg, then 0.1 mg hourly to a total of 1.0 mg in 24h	In addition to the above: nausea, vomiting, extreme brady-cardia, or development of a new arrhythmia warrants withdrawal of the drug

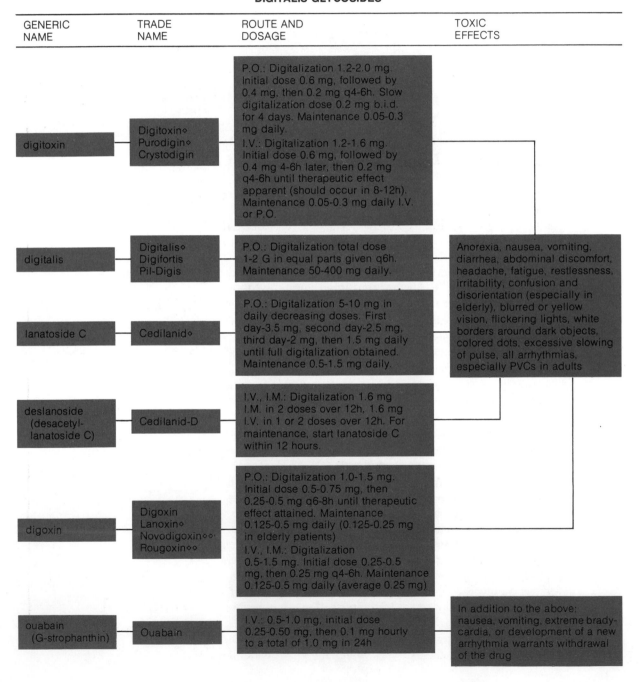

Absorption of oral digitalis glycosides is sometimes altered significantly by the conditions that are present in patients with congestive heart failure, such as vascular congestion of the enteric mucosa, hypoxia, and diarrhea.

The absorption rate also varies from one form to another. For example, the absorption rate for liquid preparations is almost 100%. But the rate for tableted digitalis glyclosides varies widely from drug to drug, and brand to brand, because of formulation differences. Given in tablet form, only 20% of lanatoside C is absorbed — compared with 40% for digitalis powder. The absorption rate for digitoxin is over 90%; the rate for digoxin is from 65% to 70%. (Ouabain, on the other hand, is absorbed so poorly and unpredictably that its oral use is not reliable.)

Naturally, any uncertainty about a drug's absorption rate makes it potentially dangerous, and this is particularly true with a digitalis glycoside. For this reason, when a patient is stabilized on one brand of tableted digitalis glycoside in the hospital, he should continue on that brand when he's discharged.

However, sometimes the doctor will switch the patient from the tableted digitalis glycosides back to oral liquid or I.V. injections of the drug. This may be necessary if the patient returns to the hospital for surgery or for treatment of a cardiac crisis. As a nurse, you should know that such a change is risky; the serum digitalis levels for I.V. injections and oral liquids of digitalis glycosides are higher than those for tableted drugs. To prevent a toxic overdose, the doctor should reduce the dosage, depending on the digitalis glycoside used.

Variations in duration of action of individual digitalis glycosides are determined mainly by the degree of plasma protein binding. Ouabain is not bound and lanatoside C is bound only slightly, which accounts for their short durations of action. In contrast, digitoxin is extensively bound to plasma protein and has the longest duration of action.

Rates of elimination of digitalis glycosides differ widely. In a matter of hours, ouabain and lanatoside C are eliminated, basically unchanged, through the kidneys, but digoxin requires approximately 36 hours for half the drug to be eliminated. Digitoxin is metabolized in the liver, excreted into the feces and (to some degree) reabsorbed into the bloodstream in a process called enterohepatic circulation. Thus, its half-life is

A guide to Canadian names
In the drug chart on the opposite page the symbol ◇ after a trade name indicates that the drug is also available in Canada. The symbol ◇◇ means that the drug is available in Canada only.

Unmarked trade names mean that the drug is available only in the United States.

The symbol G stands for gram.

These symbols will be used in all the drug charts throughout the book.

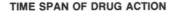

TIME SPAN OF DRUG ACTION

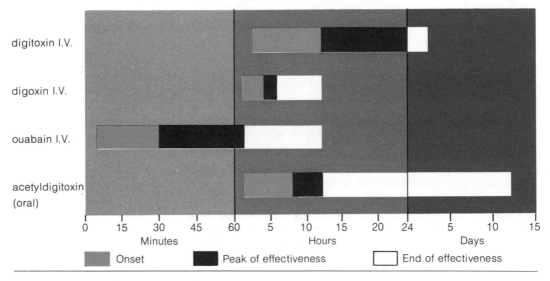

prolonged to 7 days. See the graph above for a comparison between oral and parenteral digitalization doses, as well as their rate of onset, duration of action, and rate of absorption.

Before digitalis therapy begins
Effective use of digitalis depends heavily on the doctor's clinical expertise. He completes these steps before starting digitalis.
  • First, he checks the patient for treatable disorders causing heart failure. For example, severe anemia reduces the blood's capacity to carry oxygen, and hyperthyroidism increases the tissue's demand for oxygen. Either condition may place too great a demand on the heart, causing failure. However, digitalis is not warranted in such cases, because treatment of the underlying disorder quickly eliminates the symptoms of heart failure.
  • Second, the doctor assesses the patient to determine if he will use a diuretic, digitalis, or a combination to treat him.
  • Third, the doctor assesses the severity of heart failure to determine how quickly the patient should be digitalized.
  • Fourth, he evaluates the patient's electrolyte balance,

especially the serum calcium, potassium, and magnesium levels. Abnormal levels of calcium, potassium, or magnesium increase the heart's sensitivity to digitalis, so the doctor considers this when calculating the dose and watching for signs of intoxication.

• Fifth, the doctor determines the patient's renal and liver status, because digitalis glycosides can accumulate to toxic levels if these organs are not functioning properly. For example, a patient with impaired renal function can accumulate dangerous levels of digoxin because it's mainly eliminated through the kidneys. Digitoxin, on the other hand, is eliminated mainly in the feces (and to a minor extent in the kidneys), so a dosage adjustment may or may not be needed if this drug is given to a patient with renal failure. The doctor will continue to use digoxin, but at reduced dosage. (See appendix for toxic digoxin and digitoxin serum blood levels).

• Sixth, the doctor considers the patient's total drug needs, because he knows that other drugs may increase sensitivity to digitalis. Examples are: calcium salts, which increase calcium levels; diuretics, which may cause potassium and magnesium loss; and certain steroids, which cause potassium loss and sodium retention.

After the doctor has evaluated the patient using these guidelines, he can easily choose the proper digitalis glycoside. For example, if the patient needs rapid digitalization, the doctor will probably order intravenous digoxin. It produces its full effect within one hour.

Because digoxin acts quickly, many doctors also favor it for general use. It dissipates slowly enough for stable effect, yet quickly enough to minimize the risk of toxicity.

Watching for signs of toxicity

No matter which drug the doctor chooses, you must watch every patient for signs of intoxication. All digitalis glycosides can cause them when given in high doses or for a prolonged period, though not always. As a nurse, learn to recognize them early to help prevent death from overdosage.

Some of the earliest symptoms your patient will have are extracardiac. For example, he may have gastrointestinal upsets, such as anorexia, nausea, vomiting, and abdominal discomfort. He may also report visual disturbances: blurry vision, flickering lights, yellow borders around dark objects, or

**NURSES' GUIDE TO
DIGITALIS GLYCOSIDES FOR CHILDREN**

GENERIC NAME	TRADE NAME	ROUTE AND DOSAGE	TOXIC EFFECTS
digitoxin	Digitoxin◇	Digitalization: Dose determined by age and weight, then divided into 3 or more portions and given I.V. or P.O. at 6h intervals; I.V. doses given with continuous EKG monitoring to avoid toxicity (premature/newborn — 0.022 mg/Kg; under 1 year — 0.045 mg/Kg; 1-2 years — 0.04 mg/Kg; over 2 years —0.03 mg/Kg). Maintenance: $^1/_{10}$ the digitalizing dose daily	Atrial arrhythmias most reliable and frequent signs of toxicity, whereas GI, neurologic, and visual disturbances rare as initial signs. In newborn: undue slowing of pulse, prolonged P-R interval, sinoatrial arrest.
digoxin	Digoxin◇ Lanoxin◇	P.O.: Digitalization dose determined by age and weight; initially ¼ - ½ total dose given, then ¼ total dose at 6h intervals (under 1 month — 40-60 mcg/Kg; 1 month-2 years — 60-80 mcg/Kg; 2-10 years — 40-60 mcg/Kg). Maintenance 20-30% of the digitalizing dose daily; I.M., I.V.: Digitalization dose determined by age and weight and administered in same fashion as oral preparaton (premature/newborn — 25-40 mcg/Kg; 2 weeks to 2 years — 35-50 mcg/Kg; 2-10 years — 25-40 mcg/Kg). Maintenance 20-30% of the digitalizing dose daily	

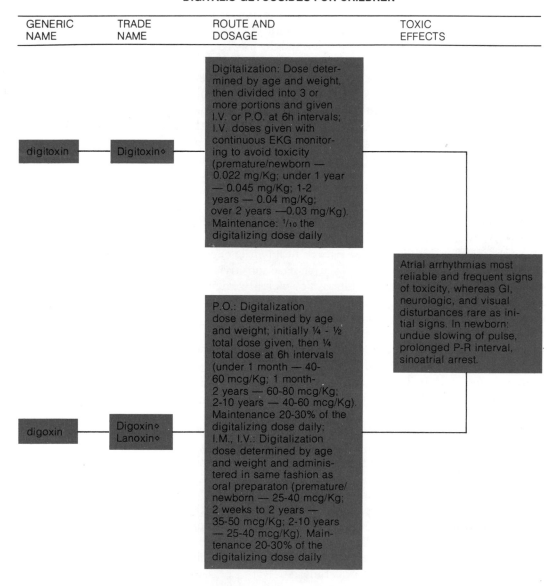

colored dots. Many patients approaching toxicity complain of restlessness, facial pain, headache, irritability, or fatigue. Elderly patients, especially, may become confused and disoriented.

Cardiac irregularities almost always develop with digitalis intoxication. In fact, they may do so without any extracardiac symptoms. You must constantly monitor patients for symptoms of irregularities, because they may precipitate pulmonary edema and cerebral or coronary insufficiency. Marked slowing of pulse rate and irregular rhythm are, in many cases, the first indications. Always check the patient's apical and radial pulse rates for one minute before administering the next dose of digitalis. Report rapid, irregular rhythm and rates below 60 in adults and 90 to 110 in children to the doctor; he may decide to withhold the drug or decrease the dosage.

Also check the patient's heart rate by EKG if you suspect a toxic arrhythmia. Digitalis overdose can produce every type of cardiac arrhythmia. The type of arrhythmia depends partly on the patient's age and other conditions, such as hypokalemia, or kidney disease. In adults, digitalis intoxication may cause premature ventricular contractions (PVCs) with possible bigeminal and trigeminal rhythms. In children, PVCs caused by digitalis are uncommon; toxicity is more likely to produce other cardiac arrhythmias.

Digitalis-induced tachyarrhythmias endanger the patient's life because they can lead to atrial or ventricular fibrillation (the most common cause of death from digitalis intoxication). To prevent a fatal arrhythmia, notify the doctor promptly anytime a patient on digitalis has an abnormal EKG.

Many disorders predispose a patient to digitalis intoxication: kidney, liver, or severe heart disease; hypokalemia; hypercalcemia; hypomagnesemia; and hypoxia. Watch any patient with these disorders closely for signs of toxicity, and check for electrolyte imbalance. If it's discovered, the doctor may then order a serum digitalis determination.

Hypokalemia is one of the most common causes of digitalis toxicity. Since potassium inhibits excitability of the heart, low serum potassium enhances ectopic pacemaker activity and possible arrhythmias.

Kidney and liver disease increase a patient's susceptibility to digitalis toxicity because (1) 60% to 80% of most digitalis glycosides are eliminated in the kidneys, and (2) most are

DRUG INTERACTIONS — DIGITALIS GLYCOSIDES

THIS DRUG	TAKEN WITH	INTERACTION
digitalis	barbiturate (phenobarbital)	Decreases digitoxin effect
digitoxin	calcium preparation (especially parenteral)	Digitalis toxicity
digoxin	amphotericin B	Digitalis toxicity, hypokalemia
	cholestyramine	Decreases digitoxin effect
	diuretics; potassium losing (Lasix, Edecrin, Hygroton, Zaroxolyn, and thiazides)	Hypokalemia, digitalis toxicity
	glucose infusion (large amounts)	Digitalis toxicity
	propranolol	Excessive bradycardia
	reserpine	Arrhythmia, especially in patients with atrial fibrillation
	antacid	Decreases digitalis absorption
	kaopectate	Decreases digitalis absorption
	sympathomimetic	Arrhythmias

inactivated in the liver. Impaired ability to excrete or inactivate digitalis causes accumulation and eventually intoxication.

Severe heart disease has the same effect as kidney or liver disease; it slows down all the body functions, allowing digitalis accumulation to toxic levels. A slowdown in body functions can also occur with age, fostering toxic reactions from small doses in elderly patients.

Many drugs interact with digitalis glycosides (see chart opposite). These interactions are dangerous for two reasons: They can precipitate toxicities and associated cardiac arrhythmias, or they can cause underdigitalization and resultant lapse into congestive heart failure.

Although the risk of drug interaction generally does not preclude the use of two agents together, you should be aware of possible complications. Take appropriate measures to monitor the patient while he's in the hospital. Then when he's discharged, warn him not to add other drugs to his regimen without his doctor's permission.

There's no specific antidote for digitalis intoxication. Treatment commonly consists of withholding digitalis until toxic symptoms have disappeared. If ventricular irritability or arrhythmias are present, other drugs may be used to speed relief, such as potassium chloride, lidocaine, procainamide, phenytoin, propranolol, or calcium-binding EDTA.

DC shock at 400 w/sec is indicated for ventricular fibrillation. It's also used for ventricular tachycardias that don't respond to drugs or are accompanied by circulatory collapse.

One further word of caution: Always double check the name and dosage of the digitalis drug before you administer it. Many are similar in spelling, though their dosage, onset, and duration of action vary greatly.

Teaching the patient about digitalis glycosides

As I described at the beginning of this chapter, many patients on digitalis therapy face a paradoxical situation. While hospitalized, they learn little about their drugs; in fact, they probably aren't even permitted to have them on their bedstands. But on the day of discharge, they are handed prescriptions for a digitalis glycoside and three or four other drugs. Suddenly they must become experts on self-administration of a complex drug regimen, and — depending on their age and emotional status — may be unable to cope with the responsibility.

You can provide the education such a patient and his family need; it should alert them to danger signs of digitalis toxicity and prompt them to seek help in time. A good way to do this is to make a patient teaching card: List the important facts he needs about his therapy in the simplest terms possible. (For a sample card, see page 43.)

Involve a relative or friend in his education to insure that he carries out instructions and calls the doctor when needed. If the patient is elderly and lives alone, arrange for a visiting nurse or check with the hospital's Social Service department. An elderly patient may be confused by a barrage of instructions, increasing the risk of overdose.

Here are the important points to teach your patient about long-term digitalis therapy:

• *Why it's needed.* Explain digitalis' action in strengthening cardiac function. Tell what is meant by a maintenance dosage and why it's required. Warn your patient not to change his dose for any reason, not to omit it on days he feels well, and not to increase it when he feels particularly ill. If he forgets to take his dose at a specified time, urge him to call his doctor. Emphasize the consequences of altering required dosages.

• *When it's toxic.* Be truthful about the dangers. Explain that digitalis has a narrow range between therapeutic and toxic effects. List these warning signs of toxicity for your patient: loss of appetite, nausea, vomiting, diarrhea, abdominal pain, headache, unusual drowsiness, disorientation, delirium, thumping feeling in chest, double vision, blurred or yellow vision, and yellow halos appearing around dark objects.

• *How other drugs interact with digitalis.* Advise the patient who requires other drugs which ones may interact with digitalis. For example, suppose a patient is taking a diuretic along with a digitalis glycoside. Explain that some diuretics are potassium wasters, and a potassium-depleted heart is more sensitive to digitalis. Because this increases his risk of intoxication (among other things), he may need a potassium supplement and he must take it as directed to avoid digitalis toxicity.

Also tell him not to take over-the-counter drugs without calling his doctor first. Many such drugs affect the action of digitalis — even cold remedies, nose drops, laxatives, and antidiarrheals.

• *How to count pulse rate.* Teach the patient to check his radial pulse, counting for at least one minute before administering his next dose. If he records a rate below 60 or notices any changes in the rate or rhythm, he should report them immediately before taking another dose.

• *How to recognize signs of congestive heart failure.* Persistent coughing, shortness of breath, and significant weight gain are early symptoms the patient can recognize. Have him weigh himself in the same clothing each day, prefer-

Dear Patient:

Here's what you should know about the drug your doctor has prescribed for you.

Digoxin regulates and strengthens your heart's pumping action so it can send needed blood to other parts of your body.

To make sure you get the most from your therapy, follow these instructions carefully.

1. Always take your pills at the *same* time each day. Take them *only* as prescribed. Never skip a dose or take extra pills without first checking with your doctor.

2. Learn to take your own pulse to record your heart's rate or rhythm. If your pulse rate is irregular, or falls below 60, call the doctor *before* you take any more pills.

3. Don't take any other drugs, including non-prescription drugs, without first asking your doctor.

Call the doctor immediately if you notice any of the following: loss of appetite, nausea, vomiting, diarrhea (for more than 1 day), change in heart rate or rhythm, blurred vision, flickering lights, yellow borders around dark objects, mental confusion, headache, or fatigue.

HOW TO TAKE YOUR PULSE
PATIENT TEACHING AID

Dear Patient:

The drug you are taking may require a periodic adjustment in dosage. To help your doctor determine when this is necessary, you must record your pulse rate and rhythm *before* you take your prescribed dose.

Here's how to take your own pulse:

1. Get a wristwatch with a second hand and place it where you can see it easily.

2. Put the fleshy part of your fingertips on the opposite wrist, in the groove just below the base of the thumb.

3. Press lightly, moving your fingertips along the groove of your wrist until you feel your pulse beat.

4. With your fingertips (never your thumb), count your pulse beat for *one minute*. Note whether it is regular or irregular. Record both rate and rhythm.

If your pulse falls below _____, or is above _____, or if it seems irregular, do not take your pills. Call the doctor immediately.

ably before breakfast. Teach him to look for signs of edema in his pretibial, ankle, and sacral areas. If any of these signs or symptoms are present, advise him to withhold his next dose of digitalis and call his doctor immediately.

• *Why dietary precautions are necessary.* Explain the need to prevent electrolyte imbalance to patients on diuretic-digitalis therapy. Reinforce any dietary instructions the doctor may have given about maintaining proper electrolyte levels.

Mr. Haines' toxic reaction: What went wrong

As you know, treating congestive heart failure frequently requires the use of one or more drugs besides the appropriate digitalis preparation. But a multiple drug regimen creates difficult problems for the doctor. He must relieve the patient's cardiac condition and at the same time avoid dangerous drug interactions.

That was the case with Mr. Haines, the 68-year-old diabetic mentioned at the beginning of this chapter. He was treated for congestive heart failure, then placed on a maintenance dosage of 0.25 mg of digoxin daily. Here is his drug regimen when he was discharged from the hospital: 0.25 mg of digoxin daily, 50 mg of hydrochlorothiazide daily, and 20 mEq of potassium chloride syrup 3 times daily. As a diabetic, Mr. Haines also continued on 0.5 gram of tolbutamide twice daily.

Three months later, Mr. Haines returned to the hospital, complaining of nausea, vomiting, abdominal pain, headache, and extreme weakness. These symptoms first appeared 3 days before. That morning, he'd awakened with diarrhea, periods of blurry vision, and mental confusion. He immediately called his family doctor, who referred him to the emergency room.

EKGs revealed that Mr. Haines was having bouts of paroxysmal atrial tachycardia, atrioventricular block, and intermittent premature ventricular contractions. These EKG findings and the gastrointestinal symptoms indicated digitalis intoxication. To obtain further confirmation, serum was drawn and sent to the lab for electrolyte measurements.

What caused this sudden intoxication? Mr. Haines had been well controlled on his drug regimen for 3 months. The doctor contacted Mr. Haines' pharmacist to check the drugs he'd been taking. The pharmacist reported that Mr. Haines was currently taking 0.25 mg of digoxin daily, 50 mg of hydrochlorothiazide daily, 0.5 gram of tolbutamide twice daily, and

20 mEq of potassium chloride 3 times daily. However, the potassium chloride prescription had not been refilled. Unless Mr. Haines had received a supply from a different pharmacist, he would not have taken any for 3 weeks.

When Mr. Haines was questioned about this later, he explained that he'd discontinued taking the potassium liquid because he could no longer tolerate its bitter, salty taste. He also volunteered that he'd been suffering from constipation and had used citrate of magnesia every other day for a month.

Initial diagnosis based on his symptoms and additional drug information was digitalis toxicity secondary to hypokalemia. The lab confirmed this diagnosis by reporting that he was slightly hyperglycemic and his serum potassium was 2.9. The hypokalemia was attributed to the potassium-depleting effect of hydrochlorothiazide and the citrate of magnesia.

Excessive use of laxatives can cause an increased loss of potassium from the bowel. In Mr. Haines' case, this loss was compounded by his discontinuing oral potassium supplement.

Digoxin and hydrochlorothiazide were held. To treat Mr. Haines' cardiac arrhythmias, we administered an I.V. of 1000 cc D_5W with 40 mEq potassium chloride to run over an 8-hour period. He also received potassium chloride syrup 20 mEq by mouth, 3 times a day. During this treatment, his EKG was constantly monitored. After 4 hours, we succeeded in controlling Mr. Haines' arrhythmias; however, we continued his I.V. until his serum potassium reached normal levels.

After 7 days with no digitalis therapy, Mr. Haines once again complained of dyspnea and other early symptoms of cardiac failure. He was redigitalized over a 2-day period with digoxin.

Mr. Haines' slight hyperglycemia was attributed to a diabetogenic effect of the hydrochlorothiazide, because he had been adequately controlled on oral therapy for 9 years. Mr. Haines needed the diuretic to help control his heart failure, so the dosage of tolbutamide was increased to 1 gram in the morning and 0.5 gram in the afternoon.

Mr. Haines responded well and remained stable for 2 days. He was discharged on the following medications: 0.25 mg of digoxin daily; 20 mEq of potassium chloride syrup 3 times daily; 1 gram of tolbutamide at 8 a.m. and 0.5 gram at 4 p.m. daily; and 50 mg of hydrochlorothiazide daily.

Before he went home this time, Mr. Haines and his family

were thoroughly counseled about his drugs. Besides this, the office nurse with Mr. Haines' family doctor was asked to check on his progress and help with his questions about medication. Mr. Haines' pharmacist was asked to monitor the drug regimen, and find a potassium chloride syrup that Mr. Haines would accept.

Fortunately, Mr. Haines has remained stable since leaving the hospital, and appears to be following his medication schedule satisfactorily. But he passed through a severe toxic reaction that could have been avoided with better instruction and monitoring by those responsible for his care.

Safe use of digitalis glycosides can be assured by only two things: adequate patient monitoring and adequate patient teaching. Both of these are partly your responsibility, as either a hospital or office nurse. You should do your share to improve the communication needed between patient, doctor, nurse, and pharmacist.

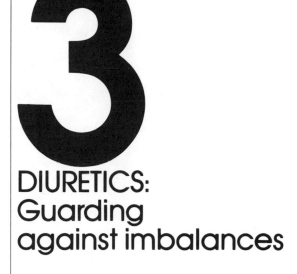

3

DIURETICS: Guarding against imbalances

BY EDMUND J. HAUGHEY, JR., PharmD
AND FRANCES M. SICA, BS

WITH THE INCREASING POPULARITY of diuretic therapy for cardiovascular problems you'll be increasingly challenged to recognize the drugs' beneficial and adverse effects. That's the impression we get in the pharmacy. Hardly a week goes by without a staff nurse calling to ask us about: the connection between diuretics and hypokalemia...between diuretics and hyperglycemia...or between diuretics and hyperuricemia.

If you work in an ambulatory setting, you're even more likely to need facts about these drugs. An office nurse told us recently about a 59-year-old patient taking between 40 and 120 mg of furosemide daily. He developed signs of hypokalemia, yet neither she nor the patient recognized them. He called her on Friday complaining of leg cramps, so she set an appointment for Monday, when the doctor would be in. By *that* time, the patient felt weak and had nausea, as well as leg cramps. If the nurse had been better informed about furosemide's action and side effects, the patient might have been spared an uncomfortable — and potentially dangerous — weekend.

How can you tell when diuretics are causing abnormal lab results or such problems as skin rash, nausea, or loss of hearing? And even if you spot the relationship, what can you

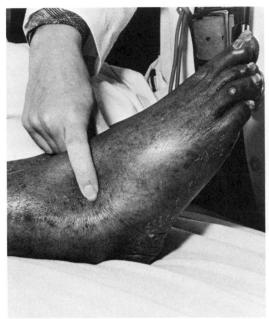 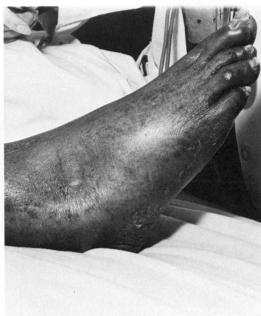

It's the pits
Pitting edema, a sign of congestive heart failure, occurs when the left ventricle lacks the strength to pump blood adequately. Extra fluid collects in the dependent part of the body, so in an ambulatory patient you'll see pitting edema in the ankle (see photos above) and in the bedridden patient, you'll see it in the sacral area.

Patients with pitting edema are treated with diuretics, given a salt-free diet, and placed on fluid restriction.

do about it? How do you answer the patient's questions? When do you call the doctor?

These are important questions. Not knowing the answers can lead to serious consequences for your patients; for example, electrolyte imbalances or even life-threatening arrhythmias. Since many doctors leave day-to-day management and patient education of diuretic therapy up to their nurses, you really must be good in two roles: as a sentinel against adverse effects, and as the patient's teacher-advisor.

How diuretics work
Diuretics differ widely in the location, strength and speed of action. To make the most of them and to stay on top of their management, you must know their whims and idiosyncrasies; that is, drug interactions that are friendly to and augment the diuretic's effects — and those that are hostile or downright inimical to good results.

Thiazide diuretics
For convenience, safety, effectiveness, and versatility, thiazides are the doctor's first choice. They affect renal tubules by inhibiting electrolyte reabsorption, particularly in

the distal tubule, thus promoting excretion of sodium and water. They're particularly useful against edema secondary to congestive heart failure, against premenstrual edema, and against drug-induced edema (secondary to steroid therapy).

They also work against edema and toxemia from pathological causes, but *not* if these conditions are associated with pregnancy.

Thiazides are also extremely valuable for controlling mild to moderate hypertension; they produce a hypotensive effect by dilating the smooth muscle of blood vessels. Initially, blood pressure falls because of decreased blood volume, but the pressure remains lowered even after blood volume returns to pre-treatment level. In many cases, thiazides alone can control hypertension but sometimes other antihypertensive drugs are needed.

Potent diuretics
Among the commercially available diuretics, two outstrip all others in potency: furosemide and ethacrynic acid.

Both act on the ascending loop of Henle to promote sodium and water excretion — but they act much more forcefully and insistently than the thiazides.

When furosemide is given for pulmonary edema, relief of pulmonary congestion comes initially from venous pooling rather than diuretic action. Within 5 minutes after I.V. administration, venous tone decreases and so does the amount of blood returning to the right atrium.

Of the two potent diuretics, furosemide gets prescribed more frequently; both, though, work well against severe edema associated with progressive congestive heart failure, or against milder edema that's unresponsive or refractory to other diuretics. They're the best diuretics for patients with renal disease, since they increase renal blood flow. They're also good for hypertension, especially if the patient also has severe edema or renal disease. Usually, they're used in combination with antihypertensives: such as, reserpine, methyldopa and guanethidine (see Chapter 6).

Potassium-sparing diuretics
Spironolactone and triamterene act on the distal segment of the kidneys to promote sodium and water excretion, but with one important difference from the other diuretics: They *block*

Check it out
Here's an important tip that will help you prevent serious, even fatal, medication errors. If you need more than one or two dosage units (ampuls, vials, tablets, and so on) to make up a single dose of any drug, check it out. You may find that the order has been transcribed incorrectly or that the decimal point was misplaced.

NURSES' GUIDE TO
COMMON DIURETICS

GENERIC NAME	TRADE NAME	ROUTE AND DOSAGE	COMMON SIDE EFFECTS

Thiazide diuretics

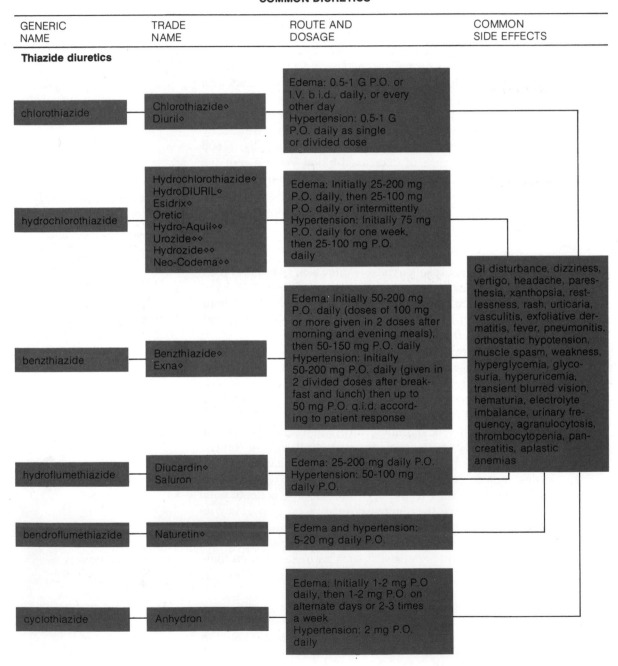

GENERIC NAME	TRADE NAME	ROUTE AND DOSAGE	COMMON SIDE EFFECTS
chlorothiazide	Chlorothiazide◊ Diuril◊	Edema: 0.5-1 G P.O. or I.V. b.i.d., daily, or every other day Hypertension: 0.5-1 G P.O. daily as single or divided dose	GI disturbance, dizziness, vertigo, headache, paresthesia, xanthopsia, restlessness, rash, urticaria, vasculitis, exfoliative dermatitis, fever, pneumonitis, orthostatic hypotension, muscle spasm, weakness, hyperglycemia, glycosuria, hyperuricemia, transient blurred vision, hematuria, electrolyte imbalance, urinary frequency, agranulocytosis, thrombocytopenia, pancreatitis, aplastic anemias
hydrochlorothiazide	Hydrochlorothiazide◊ HydroDIURIL◊ Esidrix◊ Oretic Hydro-Aquil◊◊ Urozide◊◊ Hydrozide◊◊ Neo-Codema◊◊	Edema: Initially 25-200 mg P.O. daily, then 25-100 mg P.O. daily or intermittently Hypertension: Initially 75 mg P.O. daily for one week, then 25-100 mg P.O. daily	
benzthiazide	Benzthiazide◊ Exna◊	Edema: Initially 50-200 mg P.O. daily (doses of 100 mg or more given in 2 doses after morning and evening meals), then 50-150 mg P.O. daily Hypertension: Initially 50-200 mg P.O. daily (given in 2 divided doses after breakfast and lunch) then up to 50 mg P.O. q.i.d. according to patient response	
hydroflumethiazide	Diucardin◊ Saluron	Edema: 25-200 mg daily P.O. Hypertension: 50-100 mg daily P.O.	
bendroflumethiazide	Naturetin◊	Edema and hypertension: 5-20 mg daily P.O.	
cyclothiazide	Anhydron	Edema: Initially 1-2 mg P.O daily, then 1-2 mg P.O. on alternate days or 2-3 times a week Hypertension: 2 mg P.O. daily	

NURSES' GUIDE TO
COMMON DIURETICS

GENERIC NAME	TRADE NAME	ROUTE AND DOSAGE	COMMON SIDE EFFECTS

Thiazide-like diuretics

quinethazone	Hydromox Aquamox◦◦	P.O.: 50-100 mg daily	
metalazone	Zaroxolyn◦	Edema (cardiac): 5-10 mg P.O. daily Edema (renal): 5-20 mg P.O. daily Hypertension: 2.5-5 mg P.O. daily	GI disturbance, dizziness, vertigo, headache, paresthesia, xanthopsia, restlessness, rash, urticaria, vasculitis, exfoliative dermatitis, fever, pneumonitis, orthostatic hypotension, muscle spasm, weakness, hyperglycemia, glycosuria, hyperuricemia, transient blurred vision, hematuria, electrolyte imbalance, urinary frequency, agranulocytosis, thrombocytopenia, pancreatitis, aplastic anemias
chlorthalidone	Hygroton◦ Norothalidone◦◦ Uridon◦◦	P.O.: Initially 50-100 mg daily, or 100 mg every other day then adjust maintenance dose individually	
clorexolone	Nefrolan◦◦	Edema/cardiac failure: Initially 25-50 mg P.O. on alternate days (dose may reach 100 mg), then 10-25 mg P.O. on alternate days Hypertension: Initially 10 mg P.O. daily, increased to 20 mg if necessary; in some cases, 10-20 mg P.O. on alternate days is sufficient	

Potassium-sparing diuretics

| spironolactone | Aldactone◦ | Edema: Initially 100 mg P.O. daily in divided doses, then after edema controlled, adjust dose to optimal maintenance level
Hypertension: Initially 50-100 mg P.O. daily in divided doses for at least 2 weeks, then adjust dose individually | Drowsiness, lethargy, GI distress, rash, urticaria, mental confusion, drug fever, ataxia, gynecomastia, androgenic effects including hirsuitism, irregular menses, hyperkalemia, elevated BUN |

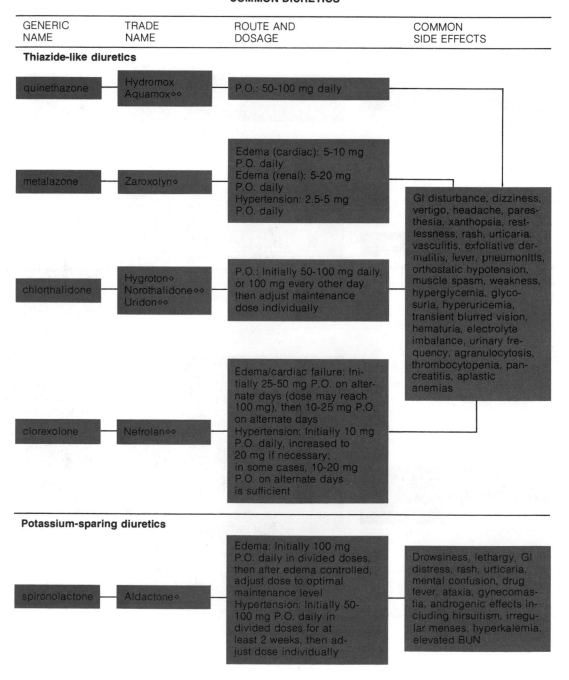

NURSES' GUIDE TO
COMMON DIURETICS

GENERIC NAME	TRADE NAME	ROUTE AND DOSAGE	COMMON SIDE EFFECTS
Potassium-sparing diuretics			
triamterene	Dyrenium◇	P.O.: 200-300 mg daily in divided doses after meals	GI distress, weakness, headache, dry mouth, rash, hyperkalemia
Potent diuretics			
ethacrynic acid	Edecrin◇	P.O.: Initially 50-200 mg daily until dry weight achieved, then reduce dosage and frequency I.V.: 50 mg, may repeat once (100 mg has been used in critical situations as a single I.V. dose)	GI disturbance, rash, dizziness, light-headedness, weakness, headache, blurred vision, fatigue, jaundice, thrombophlebitis, reversible hyperuricemia, local pain and irritation with I.V. use, dysphagia, sudden onset of watery, profuse diarrhea, ototoxicity
furosemide	Lasix◇ Furoside◇◇ Uritol◇◇ Norosemide◇◇	P.O.: 20-80 mg daily in a.m. Congestive heart failure: Initially 20-80 mg P.O., then repeat in 6-8h; if diuretic response not satisfactory, increase dose by 20-40 mg 6-8h after previous dose until satisfactory response (up to 600 mg daily in patients with severe edema) Hypertension: 40 mg P.O. b.i.d. I.M. or I.V.: 20-40 mg single dose, repeat in 2h if needed (I.V. injection should be given over 1-2 min); if diuretic response not satisfactory, increase dose by 20 mg 2h Acute pulmonary edema: 40 mg I.V. slowly, then another 40 mg 1-1½ hours later if necessary	GI disturbance, diarrhea, skin rash, dizziness, lightheadedness, weakness, headache, blurred vision, fatigue, jaundice, reversible hyperuricemia, vertigo, local pain and irritation with I.V. use, dermatitis, postural hypotension, thirst, increased perspiration, bladder spasm, urinary frequency

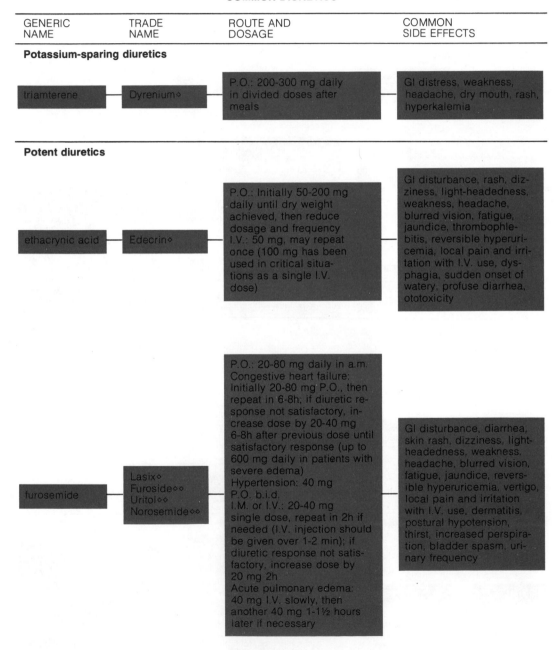

excretion of potassium, which can lead to hyperkalemia.

Although these drugs have only a mild diuretic effect, doctors value them for their ability to conserve potassium. For this reason, they're used to treat edema associated with hepatic cirrhosis and nephrotic syndrome. And they're used with other diuretics to manage hypertension and treat edema secondary to congestive heart failure. Spironolactone, administered orally, acts rather slowly. In fact, it must be continued for 3 days for maximal effect. Triamterene, administered orally, acts faster — within 2 hours — but the effect dissipates faster — within 24 hours.

Mercurial diuretics

This group once was the mainstay of potent diuretic therapy. But not today; they're rarely used because they've been replaced by safer and more effective drugs.

Teaching patients the basics

Whether you work in an office, clinic, or hospital, you have a very important job: to make the patient fully understand why he needs a diuretic. If he has a "silent" disease — say, mild hypertension — that's asymptomatic, he may decide that he doesn't need pills, at least not every day or every other day. *Convincing* him that he does need them and needs them regularly, may be very difficult. You don't want to scare him, but you must make the possible alternatives (acute MI, stroke, renal failure, and so on) clear to him. If he has congestive heart failure, make sure he understands why he's taking diuretics — to reduce body fluids, and reduce the stress on his heart.

Tell the patient that diuretic therapy isn't curative. He can't take his medications for just a few weeks or only when he's feeling "bloaty." To control hypertension or edema, he *must* take his diuretics regularly — and as prescribed.

We've overheard patients explaining to friends or relatives that they're supposed to take "one pill at breakfast" and "one pill at bedtime." Too often, all a doctor tells his patients is to take diuretics once or twice a day. Without proper counseling, patients don't understand that a pill before bed will increase their need to urinate throughout the night. For instance, a nurse told us about a 46-year-old woman who complained of insomnia while taking chlorothiazide 500 mg twice daily. If the nurse had been better informed, she'd have questioned the

POTASSIUM: THE PLUSES AND MINUSES OF BALANCE

Why such concern about potassium balance? Well, remember, potassium is the major positive charged ion in the intracellular fluid. It's vital for all cellular activities involving electrical phenomena, such as cardiac skeletal muscle contractions and the conduction of nerve impulses.

The normal serum potassium level ranges between 3.5 and 5 mEq/liter. Why and how does a potassium imbalance develop?

Hypokalemia

Most people consume from 35 to 100 mEq of potassium per day, and normally excrete 40 to 90 mEq daily in the urine, and the remainder in stools and perspiration. The body cannot conserve potassium, although it tries to maintain a high level of cellular concentration of the element: about 150 mEq/liter.

If potassium is lost without equivalent losses of protein and glycogen, the intracellular potassium decreases and true potassium deficiency occurs. If the loss continues, the patient's condition deteriorates unless intake gets adjusted and a normal level gets reestablished.

Hypokalemia (serum potassium below 3.5 mEq/liter) may be caused by a disease process (kidney disease, regional enteritis, malabsorption syndrome) ...or by drug therapy...by hormonal imbalance (excessive amounts of adrenocortical hormone)...by reduced dietary intake...by loss of gastrointestinal secretions...or by extensive burns with loss of body fluids.

Hypokalemia impairs muscle function, including respiratory muscles, causing weakness or paralysis. Impairment of smooth muscle may result in intestinal dilation and paralytic ileus.

Hypokalemia causes movement of sodium and hydrogen from extracellular fluid, excretion of hydrogen, and reabsorption of HCO_3. This leads to elevated plasma pH — metabolic alkalosis.

Hypokalemia may impair glucose tolerance, impair protein metabolism, decrease activation of certain enzyme systems, decrease water reabsorption in the renal tubule (causing polyuria or excessive excretion of urine), and produce hypocholoremic alkalosis. Cardiac effects include increased sensitivity to digitalis and ventricular extrasystoles or ventricular arrhythmias. Uncorrected, hypokalemia may lead to AV block and cardiac arrest.

Common symptoms of hypokalemia: malaise, leg cramps, arrhythmias, vomiting, dry mouth, and oliguria.

Treatment of hypokalemia

If the doctor knows of a predisposing disorder such as diarrhea, he can prevent a potassium deficit by correcting that disorder.

If hypokalemia is caused by therapy with "potassium-wasting" diuretics, it may be corrected by substituting a "potassium-sparing" diuretic such as spirono-

PATIENT TEACHING AID
POTASSIUM-RICH FOODS

MILLIEQUIVALENTS
OF POTASSIUM

FRUITS	
Apricots, raw, 2-3 medium	7.06
Banana, 1 medium	16.12
Dates, dried, 3-4	5.78
Figs, raw, fresh, 2 large	4.86
canned in syrup, 3 figs, 2 Tbsp. syrup	2.68
dried, 7 small	19.96
Oranges, 1 medium 3"	9.21
Peaches, dried, ½ cup, uncooked	28.16
Prunes, dried, raw, 5 large	7.68
Raisins, dried, seedless, 2 Tbsp.	3.68
JUICES	
Tomato, ½ cup, canned	7.29
Orange, ½ cup, fresh	5.68
MISCELLANEOUS	
Br'er Rabbit Syrup, 1 Tbsp.	6.91
5 Tbsp.	34.56
Brazil Nuts, shelled, 4 medium	2.56
shelled, ⅓ cup	17.15
Instant Coffee, Folgers, 2 G dry in 240 cc water	6.14

lactone or triamterene.

Most likely, he'll treat potassium deficiency with oral potassium supplements. Liquids such as KCl Elixir or Kaochlor are preferred, but they must be diluted with fruit juice or 8 ounces of water to avoid gastric irritation. Powdered preparations such as K-lor and K-Lyte must be dissolved, too, according to manufacturers' instructions. Liquids, powders, and the available effervescent tablets are unpalatable.

Recently, a more palatable sugar-coated tablet of potassium chloride replaced an earlier enteric-coated form which caused small bowel ulcerations. These products — Kaon-Cl and Slow-K — are in an inert wax matrix and release the drug slowly into the gastrointestinal tract, with acceptable taste and gastrointestinal safety. They're expensive, though, and require high daily dosage — 40-80 mEq/day. They're contraindicated for patients with esophageal stasis or partial obstruction (for example, from enlarged heart).

Potassium-rich foods may also correct potassium deficit, but that takes relatively large quantities and their cost is high. Many are high also in calories and sodium, and vary widely in potassium content; even the same food or drink may vary from brand to brand.

Hyperkalemia
Causes of potassium excess include inadequate renal function; adrenocortical insufficiency; potassium-sparing diuretics; and increased potassium load, as in severe tissue damage, metabolic acidosis or overtreatment with potassium salts.

Hyperkalemia means serum potassium above 5.5 mEq/liter. It may cause severe muscle weakness, paralysis, abdominal distention, diarrhea, oliguria, and anuria. Cardiac toxicity, the result of impaired conduction, is manifested by irregular ventricular rhythm. Unless the condition is reversed, ventricular fibrillation and cardiac arrest may follow.

Hyperkalemia usually gets treated by withholding potassium, "potassium-sparing" diuretics, all potassium-rich foods, and medications containing large amounts of potassium (potassium penicillin G, for example). To bind with and eliminate the ion, the doctor may order sodium polystyrene sulfonate (Kayexalate), a cation exchange resin. A common mixture is 50 gram resin suspended in 50 ml 70% sorbitol and 100 ml water administered orally via nasogastric tube or rectally. The sorbital assures passage of several loose stools daily; the excess sodium gets excreted in the stools with the potassium.

If administered rectally, this preparation should be given by high retention enema. A Foley catheter with a 30 ml balloon should be used on patients who can't retain the solution for the required length of time (preferably 4 hours). Deflate balloon in 15 minutes to avoid prolonged pressure on the rectal mucosa.

—MINNIE ROSE, RN, BS, MED

PATIENT TEACHING AID
BREAKFAST DRINKS

PRODUCT	POTASSIUM CONTENT (MG) OF RECONSTITUTED JUICE (4 OZ.)	(mEq.)
Awake, concentrate	41	1.05
Birds Eye, concentrate	232	5.93
Canned orange juice	186	4.76
Orange Plus, concentrate	254	6.50
Orange Tang (concentrate powder)	45	1.15
Fresh orange juice	200	5.11
Frozen concentrate	200	5.11

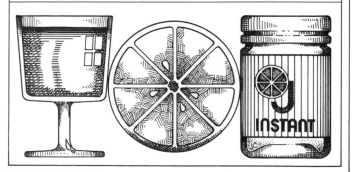

patient and discovered that she was taking her second pill late in the evening. The patient wasn't suffering from insomnia but from nocturia. An alert nurse could have solved the problem by telling the woman to take her second pill in the late afternoon.

Sometimes doctors may neglect to explain proper diet, even though they've placed a patient on salt restriction. Patients should understand that edema stems from an excess of fluid-retaining sodium in their bodies — hence, the salt restriction is a must. But they also should understand that, since diuretics cut down body sodium, they needn't go overboard by totally eliminating salt or going on an exaggerated low-salt diet.

Perhaps the most overlooked side of patient education, though, is electrolyte deficiencies. Too often patients aren't told that, in addition to ridding the body of excess sodium, many diuretics also deplete vital electrolytes — particularly potassium and chloride.

The most common, and most dangerous side effect is hypokalemia. You can learn more about this in the potassium imbalance discussion on pages 54 and 55.

The thiazides also can lead to hyponatremia, and — since they impair the kidneys' ability to clear uric acid — hyperuricemia. Hyperuricemia rarely produces symptoms and rarely leads to clinical gout, except in patients with a history of gout. If gout does develop, though, it can be controlled with a uricosuric agent.

Hyperglycemia is another side effect. No one knows exactly why this occurs — whether the thiazides affect the pancreas directly or whether hypokalemia, which suppresses insulin release, causes it. In any case, hyperglycemia usually doesn't present much of a problem, except in patients with latent diabetes or clinical diabetes. If the patient becomes symptomatic, adjusting his dose of insulin or oral hypoglycemic will control the problem.

Other side effects of the thiazides include nausea, vomiting, hypotension (especially in patients taking antihypertensive drugs), dermatologic reactions (especially in patients allergic to the sulfonamides), agranulocytosis, thrombocytopenia, pancreatitis, and aplastic anemias. If symptoms of any of these develop, the patient should see his doctor promptly.

What about the potent diuretics? Logic probably tells you that, since these drugs are called "potent" diuretics, they

DRUG INTERACTIONS — DIURETICS

THIS DRUG	TAKEN WITH	INTERACTION
chlorthalidone	corticosteroid	Induces hypokalemia
	digitalis	Causes digitalis toxicity if hypokalemic
ethacrynic acid	aminoglycoside antibiotic (Gara-mycin, Kantrex)	Increases tendency for ototoxicity
	cephaloridine	Produces nephro-toxicity
	corticosteroid	Induces hypokalemia
	digitalis	Induces digitalis toxicity if pa-tient is hypo-kalemic
furosemide	clofibrate	Increases diuretic response and mus-cular symptoms
	corticosteroid	Induces hypokalemia
	curariform drug	Potentiates curariform effects
spironolactone	potassium supplement	Induces hyperkalemia
	salicylate	Decreases diuretic effect
	thiazide	Increases diuretic effect
thiazides	cholestyramine	Decreases diuretic effect
	corticosteroid	Induces hypokalemia
	diazoxide	Induces hyperglycemia
	skeletal muscle relaxant (tubocurarine, gallamine)	Increases response to muscle relaxants

TIME SPAN OF DRUG ACTION

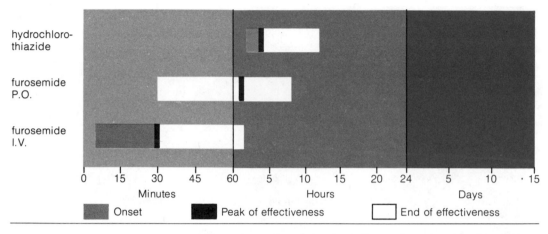

produce more dramatic side effects than the thiazides. They do — especially in the cases of hypokalemia, hyponatremia, and hypochloremia. They also may cause hypocalcemia and hypomagnesemia.

Because rapid changes in fluid and electrolyte balance may precipitate hepatic precoma or hepatic coma, potent diuretics demand caution in patients with liver disease. You should keep a sharp eye on serum potassium levels and never allow the patient to become hypokalemic.

Although I.V. administration of potent diuretics (slowly — over 1 to 2 minutes) may be just what the doctor orders for emergencies where he wants to reduce edema rapidly, it should be avoided under all other circumstances. It's been known to produce dramatic electrolyte changes, tinnitus, and deafness.

Even when given orally, potent diuretics can cause these disturbances, although usually in a milder form. The office nurse we mentioned earlier told us about a 79-year-old woman taking ethacrynic acid, 100 mg daily, who called complaining of hearing difficulties. If the nurse had been better informed, she would have recognized the hearing difficulty as a possible reaction to ethacrynic acid (ototoxicity). She would have told the patient to stop taking her medication immediately and to come in to see the doctor as soon as possible.

Potassium-sparing diuretics avoid the problem of hypokalemia, but they can cause the reverse problem —

Dear Patient:
Here's what you should know about the drug your doctor has prescribed for you. Hydrochlorothiazide removes excess water from your body so that you won't have swelling of the ankles, feet, hands, or shortness of breath. It's also used to control high blood pressure.

To make sure you get the most from your therapy, follow these instructions carefully.

1. Take your pills *only* as prescribed. Never skip a dose, increase it, or decrease it without first asking your doctor. Because your pills will increase your need to urinate, take them in the morning or before 6 p.m. to avoid unnecessary trips to the bathroom during the night.

2. Stay on the diet your doctor has given you and weigh yourself at the same time each day in similar clothing.

3. This drug may cause you to lose potassium, an *important* element in your body. If your doctor prescribes a potassium supplement to replace this loss, *be sure to take it as directed.* He may also suggest a diet rich in potassium.

4. Always tell *every* doctor who treats you that you are taking this drug.

Call the doctor immediately if you notice any of the following symptoms: dizziness, light-headedness, blurred vision, muscle cramps, fatigue, mental confusion, rash, hives, weight gain or loss of more than 5 lbs., ankle swelling, heart palpitations.

hyperkalemia — which is discussed on pages 54 and 55.

Spironolactone also can cause drowsiness, ataxia, and skin rash; triamterene also can cause headache, skin rash, and gynecomastia in males. Usually the patient can skirt gastrointestinal disturbances by taking his medications with his meals. For the other side effects, he should consult his doctor.

Recognizing toxic effects early
If you're alert to early signs of adverse drug effects, you can help by calling them to the doctor's attention. Use these checkpoints to recognize danger signals in patients:

• *Weight:* A hospitalized patient on diuretics should be weighed daily and at the same time each day before breakfast. An ambulatory patient should be weighed at every office visit. Be sure the patient wears the same clothing each time. A pronounced weight change (generally a gain or loss of 5 pounds) needs the doctor's attention.

• *Blood pressure:* This should be checked at least daily in hospitalized patients and at each office visit in ambulatory patients. Blood pressure changes may force the doctor to adjust the diuretic dosage and perhaps change any antihypertensive drugs used in combination.

• *Serum electrolytes:* As you know, diuretics can cause electrolyte disturbances, not only in potassium, but also in sodium and chloride. Hospitalized patients taking diuretics should be monitored for all electrolyte values. Ambulatory patients should be checked at least three times yearly. Patients who have renal or liver disease or who are receiving digitalis glycosides need more frequent checks.

• *Blood sugar:* If the patient has a family history of diabetes, his chances of developing hyperglycemia are particularly high. To catch it early, the doctor will order blood glucose monitored periodically.

• *Uric acid:* To detect hyperuricemia, uric acid levels should be checked on any hospitalized patient on diuretics, and at least yearly in ambulatory patients. Normal serum uric acid levels range from 2-8 mg/100 ml.

• *Renal functions:* Creatinine and blood urea nitrogen (BUN) should be checked as ordered by the doctor in all hospitalized patients, and twice a year in ambulatory patients. If the patient is high-risk, with possible renal disease, the doctor may order more frequent checks.

Make individualized care your goal

Long before now, you've learned that not all patients react to all drugs in the same way, and that any drug may produce bad side effects for some patients. But if you can teach them to take their diuretics correctly, and you can recognize side effects and drug interactions early, you can truly help them get the most from diuretic therapy.

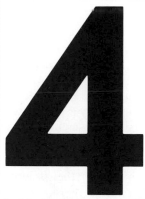

4

VASODILATORS: Making the most of anti-anginals

BY CATHERINE CIAVERELLI MANZI, RN

"I CAN'T UNDERSTAND what's wrong," gasped Mr. Stack suddenly as he was saying goodbye to departing friends. "I feel so dizzy...."

Minutes earlier, he'd slipped a nitroglycerin pill under his tongue to relieve searing anginal pain. He'd taken the same pills in the hospital, where he'd been treated several weeks earlier for angina, but this was the first time he'd used them at home. The pill relieved his pain; but now Mr. Stack had a new problem. Should he call the doctor about his dizziness? Could he afford to wait?

Cases like Mr. Stack's are not uncommon. Unfortunately, too many patients with angina have similar problems. They're discharged from the hospital with vasodilators they don't know how to take properly.

If Mr. Stack had been your patient, would you have known what to tell him about his drug? Do you know how various vasodilators work? Could you prepare a helpful teaching card? Well, this chapter will help you with these questions — and explain vasodilators in an easy-to-understand way. Then you can help patients like Mr. Stack, whose case will be concluded later in this chapter.

Introducing vasodilators

Vasodilators are life-savers for many patients suffering from coronary insufficiency. As you know, when coronary blood flow is impaired, myocardial ischemia and hypoxia may cause angina pectoris or even a life-threatening myocardial infarction. The usual cause of impaired blood supply is a narrowing of an artery or arteries from coronary atherosclerosis, vasomotor spasm, or blood clot.

During exercise or increased activity, the heart has to pump harder to get the blood and oxygen it needs. If atherosclerosis is present, this supply-and-demand ratio is altered, and ischemia of the myocardium develops — causing angina.

The goals of vasodilator drug therapy are twofold, and some drugs are used to achieve both:

• Short-term: dilation of veins and arteries (especially coronary) to increase coronary blood flow and myocardial oxygen perfusion.

• Long-term: to maintain artery dilation and enable the heart to fulfill its needs for blood and oxygen.

Vasodilators are also used with varying effectiveness to treat patients with peripheral circulatory deficiencies. And though we won't discuss them here, you will find them listed in a dosage chart in the appendices.

How they work

Although many vasodilators have long been used successfully, the way they work has not been fully determined. (I've listed the most important vasodilators in chart form on the opposite page to help you differentiate their characteristics.)

We do know what happens when nitroglycerin and other short-acting vasodilators relax (or dilate) smooth muscles in the coronary arteries and veins. This action causes pooling of blood in peripheral veins, which decreases the amount of blood flowing back to the heart. However, when the diseased heart needs an increased supply of blood — when under stress or during exercise — it can still get the increased supply without having to pump too hard, because the peripheral vascular resistance has been lowered by the vasodilator's action, further decreasing the heart's need for oxygen.

Nitroglycerin (sublingual)

Nitroglycerin is usually given sublingually and gets quickly

NURSES' GUIDE TO VASODILATORS

GENERIC NAME	TRADE NAME	ROUTE AND DOSAGE	COMMON SIDE EFFECTS
Agents for acute angina			
nitroglycerin	Nitroglycerin◇ Nitrostat◇ Nitrostabilin◇◇	Sublingual: 0.3-0.6 mg p.r.n.	Flushing, headache, postural hypotension, local burning sensation in oral cavity
isosorbide dinitrate	Isordil◇ Sorbitrate Coronex◇◇	Sublingual or slowly chewed: 2.5-5 mg p.r.n., or q2-3h P.O.: 5-30 mg q.i.d.	Flushing, headache, postural hypotension
Agents for angina prophylaxis			
nitroglycerin topical	Nitro-Bid Nitrol	Topical ointment: 1-5 inch ribbon q3-4h p.r.n. (rotate application site to prevent skin reactions)	Dermal inflammation and sensitivity, flushing, headache, postural hypotension
erythrityl tetranitrate	Cardilate◇	P.O., chewable, sublingual: 5-10 mg t.i.d. May be increased to 30 mg t.i.d.	Flushing, headache, postural hypotension, tingling sensation under the tongue (sublingual route)
mannitol-hexanitrate	Mannitol Nitranitol	P.O.: 16-64 mg q4-6h	Flushing, headache, postural hypotension
isosorbide dinitrate	Isordil◇ Sorbitrate Coronex◇◇	P.O.: 5-30 mg q.i.d., taken on empty stomach. 40 mg q6-12h (or as for acute angina)	Flushing, headache, postural hypotension, vertigo, increased intra-occular pressure
isosorbide dinitrate (sustained release)	Isordil tempids	P.O.: 40 mg q6-12h (should not be chewed)	Flushing, headache, postural hypotension, vertigo, increased intra-occular pressure
nitroglycerin (sustained release)	Nitroglycerin Nitroglyn Nitro-Bid Nitrospan Nitrong◇◇	P.O.: 1 tablet or capsule q8-12h (1.3-6.5 mg) except Nitrospan: 1 capsule q12h	Flushing, headache, postural hypotension
pentaerythritol tetranitrate (sustained release)	Pentaerythritol tetranitrate Pentritol Pentanitrol Peritrate SA◇	P.O.: 1 capsule a.m. and p.m. on empty stomach	Flushing, headache, postural hypotension
propranolol	Inderal	P.O.: 10-80 mg q6h	GI disturbance, light-headedness, rash, depression

TIME SPAN OF DRUG ACTION

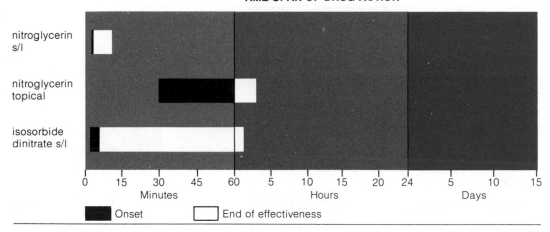

absorbed by the mucous membranes. It relieves anginal pain within one to two minutes; its level in the blood peaks in three minutes. This drug won't affect the patient's EKG patterns, but it usually causes the slight elevation in blood pressure (accompanying angina pectoris) to return to normal within 10-15 minutes.

Sublingual nitroglycerin, the drug Mr. Stack was taking, also has a short-term prophylactic effect. It may prevent an anginal attack if taken a few minutes before anticipated physical or emotional stress. Its effect lasts no more than an hour.

Caution: Nitroglycerin is contraindicated for patients with ventricular outflow obstruction, such as IHSS.

Isosorbide dinitrate

This drug is sometimes administered sublingually for short-term relief and prophylaxis for patients with coronary insufficiency. It begins to relieve pain in about 3 to 5 minutes, peaks in 15 to 30 minutes and its effect lasts 1 to 2 hours. Because isosorbide dinitrate's onset of action is slower than that of nitroglycerin, nitroglycerin is sometimes more useful for patients with acute angina.

Nitroglycerin ointment

This ointment contains 2% nitroglycerin in a lanolin-petrolatum base. When applied to the patient's skin, it gets absorbed continuously into the bloodstream and provides relief and prevention of angina attacks for 3 to 4 hours or all night (in some cases). The dosage absorbed depends on the amount of ointment applied, the area of skin covered, and the type of covering (this will be discussed later).

In the CCU, nitroglycerin ointment is used with success for patients who require constant vasodilator therapy. It can be administered even when a patient is asleep.

Propranolol
This drug is a beta adrenergic blocking drug (see Chapter 1 for how it acts on the sympathetic nervous system). Its peak effect occurs in 1 to 1½ hours and lasts for 4 hours. The drug is used to treat many patients who continue to have angina with nitroglycerin therapy (see Chapter 5).

Sodium nitroprusside
This is a pure, rapid-acting vasodilator that dilates all vascular beds (arterial more than venous) and decreases left ventricular filling pressure (preload) and decreases peripheral vascular resistance (afterload), causing increased cardiac output and decreased blood pressure. It prevents further ischemic heart damage with acute myocardial infarction.

Nitroprusside is a reddish-brown powder that must be dissolved in D_5W before administration. Because this preparation is light-sensitive, the container and I.V. tubing must be wrapped in foil and black tape. (For a photo showing how this is done, see Chapter 10.) Do not keep the solution longer than 4 hours.

Nitroprusside is administered only by slow infusion in a hospital where the patient can be properly monitored. An infusion pump, micro-drip regulator, or similar device is needed to insure exact regulation of the flow rate.

Cyanide is formed as nitroprusside interacts with red blood cells and body tissue. A liver enzyme called rhodanase transforms the cyanide to thiocyanate, which (in toxic levels) can cause serious side effects. Toxicity of thiocyanate begins at plasma levels of 5-10 mg/100 ml of blood. Fatalities at levels of 20 mg/100 ml have been reported.

When a patient is taking nitroprusside, his thiocyanate serum levels should be drawn every 72 hours as long as he is on the drug. Suspect thiocyanate toxicity if the patient develops these symptoms: nausea, anorexia, disorientation, muscle spasms,

DRUG INTERACTIONS — VASODILATORS

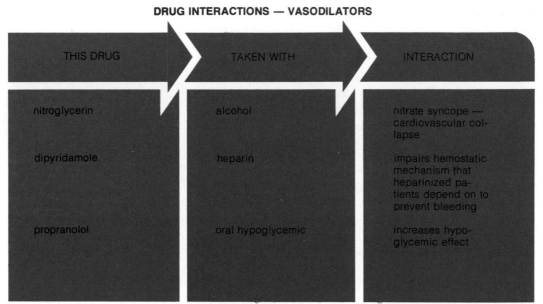

THIS DRUG	TAKEN WITH	INTERACTION
nitroglycerin	alcohol	nitrate syncope — cardiovascular collapse
dipyridamole	heparin	impairs hemostatic mechanism that heparinized patients depend on to prevent bleeding
propranolol	oral hypoglycemic	increases hypoglycemic effect

or psychotic behavior. Tissue anoxia is also present and may lead to metabolic acidosis.

Evaluating patients
Take a thorough history — that's your first job in evaluating a patient who might benefit from vasodilator therapy or who's already on vasodilators and still suffers. A patient with angina pectoris will usually describe his symptoms in glowing detail, if you encourage him to talk freely and in his own words. His description of the pain — and the pattern it follows — is the key to evaluation.

He'll probably describe his pain with words such as "strangling," "squeezing," "pressing," "burning," "choking," or "bursting." Typically the pain starts in the anterior area of the patient's chest and may radiate to his left shoulder and down his arm. Some patients experience a numbness or weakness in arms, wrists, or hands, as well as feelings of great apprehension and impending death. Many patients involuntarily clutch one or both of their clenched fists over the site of the pain. The patient's suffering may force him to lie down and rest.

Angina usually stems from an emotional or physical stress and it subsides quickly when the patient rests.

But, some anginal attacks do occur while the patient is resting. These attacks usually last 10 to 15 minutes. If the pain lasts longer than 30 minutes — or is unrelieved by 3 pills taken 10 minutes apart — he should be warned he may be having a myocardial infarction. If the pain is relieved in about 3 minutes by sublingual nitroglycerin, the chances are good the patient is suffering only from angina.

Ask the patient specifically what drugs he might be taking — when and how much. Many angina sufferers will already be on vasodilators, and the doctor must be advised of this. Look for any mistakes the patient might be making in taking his drugs.

Unlike most anginal episodes, a myocardial infarction may begin suddenly while the patient is at rest. You've probably learned to recognize the symptoms — shortness of breath and extremely oppressive pain under the lower part of the patient's sternum. His pulse may be rapid and weak and perhaps irregular. He may become nauseous and show some of the symptoms of shock — paleness, cyanosis, cold, clammy skin, and low blood pressure.

Why patient teaching is needed

Unfortunately, many doctors start patients on vasodilators with little more instruction than, "Take one under your tongue when you have heart pain." This is all Mr. Stack was told, which is why he was surprised by his attack of dizziness.

Properly taught, he would have been warned that nitroglycerin can cause postural hypotension. He should sit or lie down for several minutes after each dosage to prevent this from happening. Naturally, Mr. Stack found this out when he called his doctor. But the episode could have been better understood with proper teaching.

Other misunderstandings about vasodilators cause equally distressing problems for patients. For example, some patients get the odd notion that prophylactic vasodilators are addictive. Others think, "If one pill relieves the pain, five pills ought to cure me completely." You'll often be in the best position to identify the patient's misunderstandings and provide him with the information he needs.

A good way to begin is to give the patient a teaching card that explains what his disorder is, how the drug will benefit him, and how he should take it. Then you could tell him something like this: Your heart muscle isn't getting the amount

NITROGLYCERIN
PATIENT TEACHING AID

Dear Patient:
Here's what you should know about the drug your doctor has prescribed for you.
Nitroglycerin relieves anginal pain by temporarily dilating (widening) veins and arteries. This brings more blood and oxygen to the heart when it needs it most, and your heart doesn't have to work so hard.

To make sure you get the most from your therapy, follow these instructions carefully:

1. When you get anginal pain, stop what you are doing, lie down, and put a pill under your tongue. Let it dissolve completely and hold the saliva in your mouth for 1 to 2 minutes before swallowing. Always sit or lie down when you take your pill or you may get dizzy. If you feel headachy or your face flushes after taking your pill, don't worry. These effects are only temporary.

2. Take up to 3 pills — one every ten minutes — for pain. Record each dosage. *If the pain doesn't go away after 30 minutes, or is unusually severe, call the doctor at once or go to the hospital emergency ward.*

3. Don't drink alcohol without asking your doctor first.

4. Never stop taking your pills altogether without your doctor's permission. However, don't worry about taking them as needed because they are not habit-forming.

5. Keep your pills in their original container with the cotton removed. They will lose their strength if they're exposed to light, moisture, or heat — or if they're more than 3 months old. Get fresh ones after 3 months. Fresh pills produce a slight burning sensation under your tongue.

Call the doctor immediately if you notice any of the following: unusually severe or prolonged pain, fainting, or dizziness.

of blood it needs. These drugs will help prevent the heart from being overworked. If it does become overworked and causes anginal pain, the drugs will help relieve the pain.

Many patients don't understand "sublingual," so tell them specifically to place a sublingual tablet under their tongue and allow it to completely dissolve. To maintain maximum effect, they should hold the saliva in their mouth for 1 to 2 minutes before swallowing.

Caution specifically against overdosage. (This is a danger even in a hospital where the patient may have nitroglycerin pills at his bedside. Tell the patient to report each dose so it can be charted.) At home, the patient should immediately contact his doctor if he feels no relief after 3 doses, because he might be developing a myocardial infarction. Occasionally the lack of relief may be caused by the drug's loss of potency. If the patient does not experience a burning sensation or get a bitter taste when he takes his nitroglycerin, the pill has probably lost some of its potency.

Also caution the patient never to discontinue his vaso-

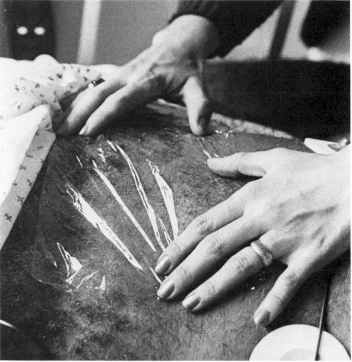

dilators without first checking with his doctor, because of the
chance of serious withdrawal effects. For example, if propranolol were discontinued suddenly, a rebound phenomenon
could occur, increasing the frequency and severity of the
anginal attacks, and possibly precipitating myocardial infarction.

Another caution: *Alcohol and vasodilators don't mix.* If the
patient takes nitroglycerin after imbibing, the result may be a
nitrate syncope (sudden loss of consciousness from decreased
blood supply to the brain).

Make sure the patient understands that nitroglycerin tablets
lose their effectiveness quickly, especially when exposed to
heat, light, or moisture. He should keep them in their *original*
container (with the cotton removed) and never carry them in a
pocket close to body heat. To make sure the patient has potent
drugs, tell him to get a fresh supply every 3 months, even if he
still has tablets left.

Patients who'll be using nitroglycerin ointment need special
instructions. They can apply the ointment to any part of skin

that's fairly free of hair. Many patients prefer the chest for psychological reasons, because that's where the anginal pain originates.

Have the patient practice measuring the dose with the ruled paper that's packed with the drug. Then show him how to spread it onto his skin in a 6-inch circle.

Some manufacturers recommend taping the ruled filter paper over the anointed area to keep the ointment from rubbing off. However, I teach my patients to use a piece of Saran Wrap. It stays in place better, leaks less ointment, and decreases skin irritation. But it also increases the amount of ointment absorbed — a good reason never to vary the type of covering used, once dosage is established. Another important point: When *you* apply the ointment, never get it on your skin, lest *you* absorb it.

Sending the patient home

By knowing what to tell patients about vasodilators, you'll be able to reassure them greatly — and protect them. When angina pain strikes, they'll know what to do and what effects to expect. You'll help keep them from unnecesary discomfort and perhaps save a life.

5

ANTIARRHYTHMICS: Being prepared with the right drugs

BY MICHAEL R. COHEN, BS Pharm

"MY HEART'S SKIPPING BEATS," said 48-year-old Mr. Wiedman apprehensively, when the nurse asked how he felt.

The scene was a surgical unit, where Mr. Wiedman had been recovering well from a hernia operation. That evening he looked pale, however, so the nurse immediately took his radial pulse; it was rapid and irregular. She then checked his apical pulse; it was 170/min. His blood pressure was 90/70. Earlier that day it had been 118/70.

The nurse called the doctor. She knew that Mr. Wiedman had a myocardial infarction 4 years before. He'd been taking quinidine and propranolol which were discontinued before surgery. But, what did she do next? What drugs should you have ready when a patient develops an arrhythmia? What special equipment will the doctor need? How can you prevent the patient's condition from becoming more serious?

Dangerous arrhythmias don't happen exclusively in the CCU, you know. They can also occur in a medical/surgical unit...or anyplace. That's why you need to understand how antiarrhythmic drugs are used, how they're administered, their interactions, and their side effects.

Six drugs are currently in use; you'll find them discussed in

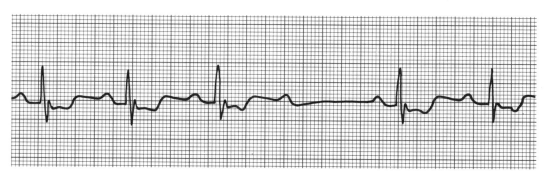

Heart block
An early sign of quinidine toxicity is a second-degree AV heart block. The EKG shows a QRS complex dropped after a P wave, a constant P-P interval, and an unvarying P-R interval.

this chapter. They are quinidine, procainamide, disopyramide, lidocaine, phenytoin, and propranolol. By learning how they work, you'll be better able to assist the doctor by having the right drugs ready in an emergency.

Quinidine

Quinidine is the drug of choice for treating premature atrial contractions (PACs) and preventing atrial fibrillation, but it has been largely replaced by electrical cardioversion for converting atrial fibrillation to normal sinus rhythm. It's effective in treating atrial flutter, but the patient should be digitalized first to avoid possible increased ventricular rate due to slowed atrial activity and enhanced atrioventricular conduction. Quinidine is also very effective for premature ventricular contractions, but may not be the drug of choice for supraventricular tachycardias. It can be combined with propranolol in treating paroxysmal atrial arrhythmias when propranolol alone has been ineffective.

Three salts of quinidine are available: sulfate, gluconate, and polygalacturonate. The sulfate salt is the cheapest and produces the fastest, shortest effect. The gluconate and polygalacturonate, supposedly better tolerated, are usually prescribed for patients who experience nausea and vomiting after taking the sulfate. In emergencies, quinidine gluconate might be given intramuscularly. I.V. administration is not recommended because it has caused so many toxic reactions: notably hypotension and prolonged QRS and QT intervals. Instead, procainamide is preferred for I.V. use.

Quinidine can, in sufficient doses, depress myocardial excitability enough to cause cardiac arrest. You must be particularly alert to this possibility in patients with heart failure or liver or kidney disease because such conditions interfere with metabolism and excretion of quinidine, resulting in higher drug concentrations in the body. The EKG gives early evidence of toxicity: prolonged QRS complexes, evidence of second degree or complete heart block, or premature ventricular contractions — all require discontinuing quinidine.

Many drugs interact with quinidine. As an anticholinergic, it antagonizes the effects of cholinergic drugs, such as bethanechol and pilocarpine. For example, it tends to prevent the cardiac slowing produced by cholinergic drugs; therefore, in a patient receiving cholinergic drugs, it may fail to terminate paroxysmal supraventricular tachycardia. Conversely, quinidine has an additive effect with anticholinergic agents (atropine, belladonna, dicyclomine, propantheline).

Quinidine may produce additive hypoprothrombinemic effects with the coumarin anticoagulants, so closely observe patients taking anticoagulants with quinidine. However, the risk of hemorrhage is not high.

Intravenous quinidine (or high oral or I.M. doses) can cause sufficient vasodilation to reduce blood pressure significantly. So watch for possible additive hypotensive effect in patients taking quinidine with antihypertensive drugs.

Quinidine potentiates both non-depolarizing and depolarizing muscle relaxants, so giving it to a patient who has been given curare or succinylcholine may cause unresponsiveness and apnea. In fact, quinidine is best avoided in the immediate postoperative period when the effects of muscle relaxants may still be present. Quinidine may antagonize the effects of neostigmine and edrophonium, used to treat myasthenia gravis.

Quinidine and digitalis have several opposing cardiac effects. Quinidine slows atrial conduction; while digitalis speeds conduction. Digitalis strengthens muscular contraction; quinidine may counteract this effect. However, sometimes they are used together.

Quinidine is *absolutely contraindicated* in cases of second- or third-degree heart block. *Be especially watchful of this should a patient have digitalis toxicity.*

Procainamide

Procainamide is most commonly used to treat premature ventricular contractions or ventricular tachycardia and is occasionally used to treat supraventricular arrhythmias after quinidine has failed. It may be given to patients who cannot

NURSES' GUIDE TO
ANTIARRHYTHMICS

GENERIC NAME	TRADE NAME	ROUTE AND DOSAGE	COMMON SIDE EFFECTS
quinidine	Quinidine sulfate◇ Quiniglute dura-tabs◇ Cardioquin◇ Biquin◇◇ Quinate◇◇	P.O.: Test dose of 1 tablet to determine idiosyncrasy, then 200-300 mg q4-6h	Tinnitus, headache, nausea, disturbed vision, cardiac asystole, ventricular ectopic beats, idioventricular rhythms, paradoxical tachycardia, vomiting, diarrhea, abdominal pain, vertigo, excitement, confusion, cutaneous flushing with intense pruritus
	Quinidine gluconate	I.M.: Initial dose 375-400 mg then 200 mg q2h, times four (for acute tachycardia) I.V.: 330 mg or less to maximum of 750 mg (diluted in 50 ml 5% glucose at rate of 1 ml/min)	
procainamide hydrochloride	Procainamide◇ Pronestyl◇	P.O.: 250-500 mg q3-4h I.M.: 0.5-1.0 G q6h until oral preparation feasible I.V.: Bolus 50-100 mg. Drip 1-2 amps in 500 cc D₅W 1-4 mg/min	I.V., I.M.; hypotension, serious disturbances of cardiac rhythm. Anorexia, nausea, urticaria, pruritus, lupus erythematosus syndrome, fever, chills, diarrhea, weakness, depression, psychosis.
lidocaine hydrochloride	Lidocaine◇ Xylocaine◇	I.V.: Bolus 50-100 mg — may repeat in 5 min. No more than 200-300 mg in 1 hour Continuous infusion: 1-2 G in 500 ml D₅W at 2-3 mg/min I.M.: 4.3 mg/Kg weight, injected into deltoid muscle, may repeat in 60-90 minutes (rare)	Drowsiness, dizziness, tinnitus, visual disturbances, vomiting, sensations of cold, or numbness, twitching, convulsions, hypotension, cardiovascular collapse, bradycardia, depression, confusion, slurred speech, agitation
propranolol hydrochloride	Inderal	P.O.: 10-40 mg q.i.d. up to 400 mg per day I.V.: 1-3 mg (I.V. use only for life-threatening arrhythmias)	Bradycardia, congestive heart failure, intensification of AV block, hypotension, light-headedness, visual disturbances, disorientation, GI distress, bronchospasm
disopyramide phosphate	Norpace Rhythmodan◇◇	P.O.: 100-150 mg q6h	GI distress, dry mouth, pruritus, urticaria, headache, pallor, confusion, fatigue, insomnia, urinary retention
phenytoin phenytoin sodium	Dilantin◇ Diphenyl Novophenyl◇◇ Dantoin◇◇	P.O.: 100-200 mg q.i.d. I.V.: 500 mg-1 G slow I.V. push, not to exceed 50 mg/min	GI disturbances, fever, nystagmus, ataxia, slurred speech, diplopia, depression, tremor, headache

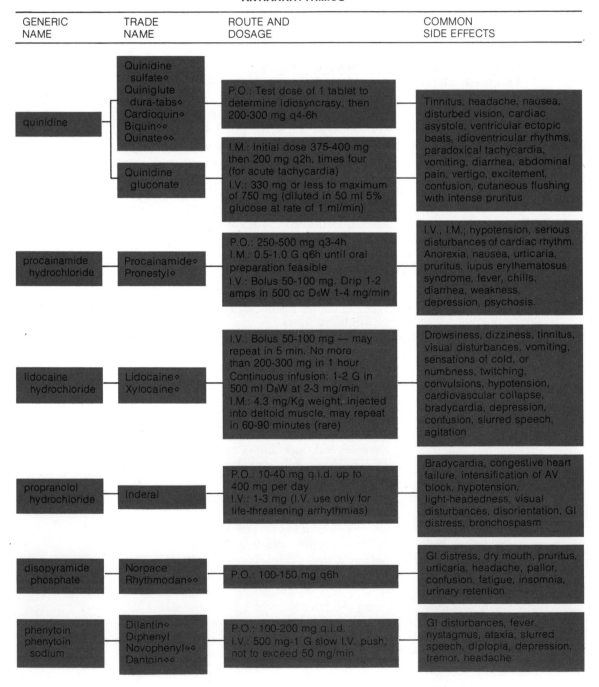

tolerate or who are sensitive to quinidine. Also, it may be given with quinidine.

Procainamide's effects on the heart are similar to those of quinidine. For years it played second fiddle to quinidine, but has been used more lately because of quinidine's scarcity and rising cost. Its side effects, too, are similar to those of quinidine: hypotension, (especially severe after I.V. administration), anorexia, nausea and vomiting. It has also produced a syndrome resembling lupus erythematosus, characterized by fever, arthralgia, erythema, and scaling of the skin. The syndrome is usually reversible once the drug is discontinued.

Procainamide toxicity is shown by a prolonged QRS complex and QT interval. In very large doses it causes degrees of heart block with a prolonged P-R interval.

Procainamide is partially metabolized after absorption by the GI tract and then it's excreted by the kidneys; therefore, you have to carefully monitor its use in patients in renal failure or patients with decreased renal blood flow.

Procainamide's interactions are also similar to quinidine: enhancing the effect of antihypertensives, especially when administered parenterally, and enhancing the effects of other anticholinergic drugs while antagonizing those of cholinergic drugs. Procainamide may potentiate the neuromuscular blocking drugs and should be used with caution after surgery.

Procainamide can be administered orally, intramuscularly and intravenously, but I.V. administration is rare now that lidocaine is available. When procainamide is given intravenously, EKG and blood pressure monitoring are required. Notify the doctor if you see such EKG danger signs as widening of the QRS complex. Be prepared to administer a vasopressor agent such as levarterenol or dopamine if hypotension develops.

Disopyramide

Disopyramide is a new oral antiarrhythmic drug. It was approved for use in the United States in September 1977, and in Canada a few months earlier. So far its use is limited to treating multifocal, unifocal, and paired premature ventricular contractions and episodes of ventricular tachycardia. It is effective in both digitalized and nondigitalized patients.

Clinical studies now under way may extend its use. Disopyramide is being studied in patients with myocardial infarctions, atrial arrhythmias, heart failure, and severe conduction disturbances. It is being studied for interactions with beta blockers and other drugs. Also, an I.V. form is being studied.

Obviously, clinical experience with disopyramide is limited, yet in clinical trials it did appear to have fewer severe side effects than quinidine sulfate, the standard against which it was tested. For instance, disopyramide produced less nausea, vomiting, diarrhea and fever. Its most common side effects were dry mouth and urinary retention. This drug is contraindicated for patients in cardiogenic shock.

Lidocaine

Lidocaine is the drug of choice for ventricular arrhythmias following acute myocardial infarction and for ventricular tachycardia, including those cases caused by digitalis toxicity. It has been used for prophylaxis and for the treatment of ventricular arrhythmias after cardioversion. It is not effective against most supraventricular rhythms.

Lidocaine is administered intravenously. The initial bolus dose of 100 mg is followed by constant infusion of 2 to 3 mg/min, adjusted by monitoring with EKG. (See the graph in Chapter 9 for an explanation of why this is done). Lidocaine produces its effect rapidly and is rapidly cleared from the bloodstream. Thus, side effects are of brief duration.

Lidocaine's major side effects: central nervous system disturbances such as depression, confusion, dizziness, disorientation, diplopia, stupor and convulsions. Convulsions can be controlled with diazepam, 5 to 10 mg I.V. Other side effects include muscle twitching, agitation, hearing loss, paresthesia and respiratory and circulatory depression. Excessive doses can slow an already damaged heart, resulting in hypotension and pulmonary congestion.

Phenytoin

Phenytoin (formerly diphenylhydantoin) is being used in some hospitals to treat certain cardiac arrhythmias, especially those caused by digitalis toxicity. The initial dose, 500 mg to 1 gram by slow I.V. push, is followed by an I.V. or oral maintenance dose of 300 to 400 mg per day. However, I.V. use reportedly has caused hypotension, shock, respiratory and cardiac arrest in some cases. Phenytoin is not ordinarily given as a continuous I.V. drip because it crystalizes in available diluent solu-

DRUG INTERACTIONS — ANTIARRHYTHMICS

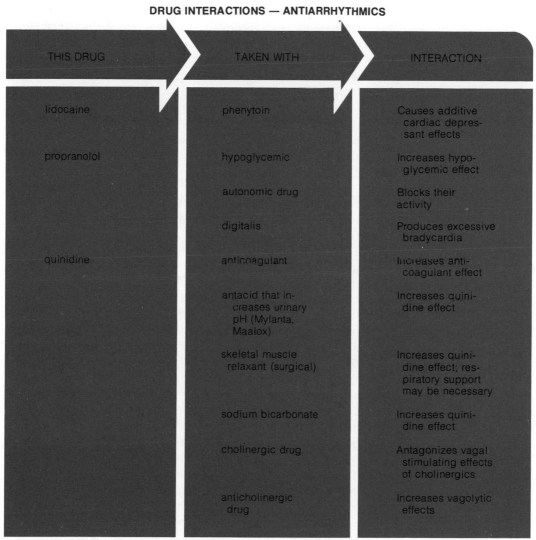

THIS DRUG	TAKEN WITH	INTERACTION
lidocaine	phenytoin	Causes additive cardiac depressant effects
propranolol	hypoglycemic	Increases hypoglycemic effect
	autonomic drug	Blocks their activity
	digitalis	Produces excessive bradycardia
quinidine	anticoagulant	Increases anticoagulant effect
	antacid that increases urinary pH (Mylanta, Maalox)	Increases quinidine effect
	skeletal muscle relaxant (surgical)	Increases quinidine effect; respiratory support may be necessary
	sodium bicarbonate	Increases quinidine effect
	cholinergic drug	Antagonizes vagal stimulating effects of cholinergics
	anticholinergic drug	Increases vagolytic effects

tions. (Some doctors may still prescribe I.V. drip. When they do, phenytoin should be diluted with normal saline, never in dextrose solution or the drug will separate from the solution.)

Propranolol

Propranolol is most valuable in treating atrial arrhythmias. It reduces the ventricular response to atrial flutter and fibrillation and is effective when ventricular rates cannot be controlled by digitalis. It may also make supraventricular tachycardia more responsive to vagal stimulation. It reduces or abolishes atrial tachycardia. Propranolol does not inhibit digitalis' inotropic action; hence the two drugs constitute an effective combination in treating patients with ventricular failure (see Chapter 2).

Bradycardia is a dangerous side effect of propranolol, especially in patients with myocardial damage. It can sometimes be successfully treated with atropine or isoproterenol. Hypotension and increased airway resistance are other side effects, so carefully monitor patients with pulmonary disease.

Propranolol must always be withdrawn gradually. Studies show that sudden withdrawal can cause a dangerous rebound reaction *in patients with unstable angina pectoris*. The reaction begins with anginal pain of increasing frequency and severity sometimes followed by myocardial infarction, ventricular arrhythmias and death.

Always warn outpatients that they must not suddenly discontinue the drug — that it must be withdrawn over 2 weeks or more. If side effects develop requiring prompt withdrawal, the patient should be hospitalized for close observation. If he develops angina, propranolol may have to be reinstituted and then tapered off gradually.

Many drugs interact with propranolol because of its beta-adrenergic blocking and other pharmacologic activities (see Chapter 1). It blocks isoproterenol, a beta adrenergic stimulant, so the two should not be used together. Propranolol's beta adrenergic blocking activity may potentiate the action of reserpine and other catecholamine-depleting drugs. Caution: This drug is contraindicated for patients with asthma.

Propranolol must be used cautiously for treating digitalis-induced arrhythmias, because it may potentiate the bradycardia caused by digitalis. Propranolol's antihypertensive action may cause excessive hypotension when combined with such agents as guanethidine, methyldopa and hydralazine, so patients should be monitored closely when on widely used combined therapy.

Propranolol may potentiate the hypoglycemic effect of insulin and the oral agents and may mask hypoglycemic reactions by preventing sweating and tachycardia, cardinal signs of acute hypoglycemia.

The oral dose of propranolol is 10 to 40 mg, 3 to 4 times daily,

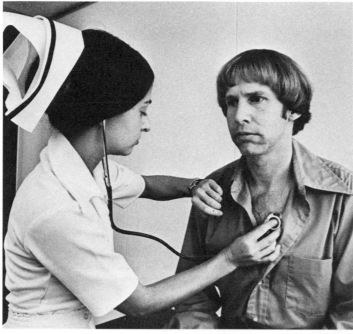

Watch the beat
Anytime you feel an irregular rhythm in the radial pulse, check the apical pulse for one minute and compare the difference in rate. This is called a pulse deficit. It may indicate weak ventricular contractions and serious arrhythmias. If the pulse deficit exceeds 10, call the doctor.

before meals and at bedtime. Higher doses are necessary for angina and hypertension. The intravenous dose is 1 to 3 mg, given while monitoring the effect by EKG. Atropine should be on hand for correcting excessive bradycardia. The substantial difference in oral and intravenous doses stems from the fact that oral propranolol is broken down in the liver before it produces its effect. Occasionally, a patient is shifted from the oral to the I.V. route. If this is ordered without adjusting the dose, you should withhold the drug. An I.V. dose of 10 to 40 mg could cause death.

Assessment on a medical/surgical unit
Admittedly, those of you working on medical/surgical units lack the equipment and staff that are available in a CCU. But you do have your sight, hearing, and touch; most important, you have a mind trained to interpret your observations. You can and should detect most serious cardiac rhythm abnormalities and intervene effectively. See *Nursing Skillbook,* ASSESSING VITAL FUNCTIONS ACCURATELY, Chapters 1 and 6.

Always be sure to identify the cardiac patients on your unit — no matter what their current diagnoses may be. Any patient

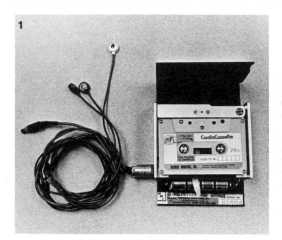

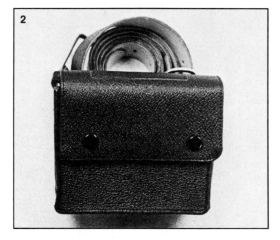

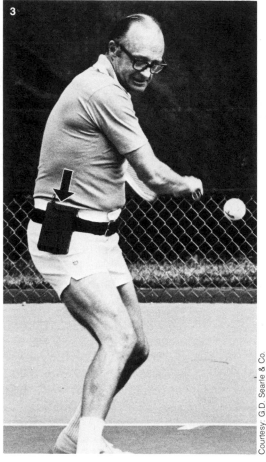

Holter to health

Ambulatory electrocardiography, also known as Holter monitoring after Dr. Norman J. Holter who conceived and developed the process, enables a doctor to monitor as many as 100,000 cardiac cycles over a 24-hour period. The advantages of this method are many.

With very little equipment, the doctor can hook up a patient to one or more EKG leads. These record onto a portable cassette tape recorder (Figure 1) which the patient can wear easily on his belt (Figure 2).

The recorder should be connected to an EKG for test readings. After the hookup has been checked, the patient goes through a normal day (Figure 3) on the monitor. He is encouraged to try out those activities that bring on his symptoms, keeping a diary to record the exact times of symptoms, activities, and any drugs he takes so that their impact can be correlated with the EKG printouts. With the aid of a high-speed scanner (Figures 4 and 5), the doctor can review 24 hours of tape in 24 minutes, picking up important EKG changes.

Although not a substitute for CCU monitoring, the Holter monitor can catch a sporadic rhythm disturbance that an office or stress-test EKG might miss. It also saves the patient the time and expense of a hospital stay.

Holter monitoring has proved useful for patients recuperating from myocardial infarctions, those taking antiarrhythmic drugs, or those using pacemakers. It can catch rate, rhythm, and conduction abnormalities as well as cardiac responses to a normal environment. It is especially useful in diagnosing arrhythmias and CNS symptoms such as dizziness, syncope, and pain.

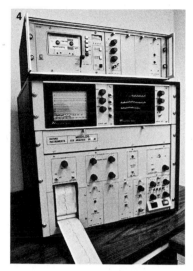

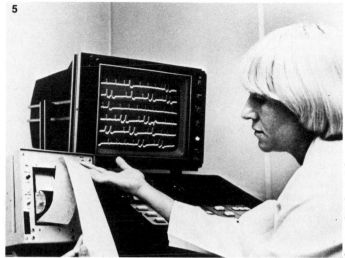

Courtesy: G.D. Searle & Co.

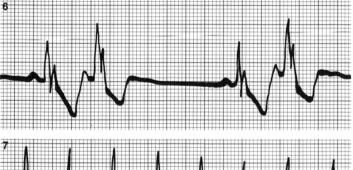

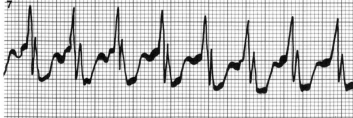

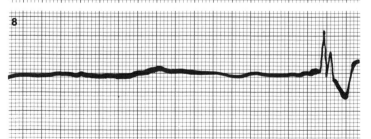

Sick at heart

When Joshua Burle, a 62-year-old accountant began complaining of dizzy spells, his doctor performed an EKG in the office. He found nothing of significance. So he put Mr. Burle on a 24-hour Holter monitor. The EKG printouts to the left show a portion of what the doctor found.

Figure 6, recorded at 3:45 a.m., shows Mr. Burle experiencing sinus bradycardia with PVCs while he slept. Note the compensatory pause following the ectopic ventricular beats.

Figure 7, recorded at 4:05 a.m., shows Mr. Burle in supraventricular tachycardia. His ventricular rate at this time was 136-150/min. Note that the R-R interval is slightly irregular.

Figure 8, recorded at 4:06 a.m., shows Mr. Burle going into asystole for nine seconds.

The full 24-hour monitoring revealed frequent periods of asystole. With the Holter monitor, Mr. Burle's doctor was able to identify the cause of the dizzy spells as hypoxia. He ordered further tests including cardiac catheterization, which confirmed a diagnosis of aortic stenosis.

PROPRANOLOL
PATIENT TEACHING AID

Dear Patient:

Here's what you should know about the drug your doctor has prescribed for you.

Propranolol helps your heart by slowing and regulating its beat. This decreases the amount of blood and oxygen your heart needs and lightens its workload.

To make sure you get the most from your therapy, follow these instructions carefully:

1. Always take your pulse rate before each dosage. If it falls outside the range your doctor gives you, *call him before you take another dose.*

2. If you are a diabetic, be sure to tell the doctor. This drug may hide the signs and symptoms of low blood sugar.

3. *Never discontinue taking this drug without instructions from your doctor.* This can be very dangerous.

Call the doctor immediately if you notice any of the following: wheezing or shortness of breath, depression, ankle swelling, fatigue, weakness, dizziness, weight gain greater than 2 lbs in 1 day or 7 lbs in 1 week, insomnia, rash, diarrhea, or constipation.

PROCAINAMIDE
PATIENT TEACHING AID

Dear Patient:

Here's what you should know about the drug your doctor has prescribed for you.

Procainamide helps your heart by wiping out those unnecessary extra beats, which you may or may not have noticed.

To make sure you get the most from your therapy, follow these instructions carefully:

1. Because procainamide can sometimes cause stomach distress, take your pills with milk or a meal.

2. *Take your pills only as prescribed.* This drug must be taken at regular intervals *on schedule.*

Call your doctor immediately if you notice any of the following: prolonged nausea or vomiting, heart palpitations, rash, hives, chills, fever, dizziness, vision problems, aching muscles or joints, or chest pain when you take a deep breath.

with a history of a myocardial infarction or other coronary disease deserves extra attention. Make sure to look in on him several times each shift, even though you're busy. Be alert for signs and symptoms suggesting abnormal rhythm, and check them out promptly.

Three observations are particularly meaningful:

• *Heart rate:* Use your stethoscope. Check the apical pulse every time you check the radial (see page 79). If there's a difference, subtract to determine the pulse deficit, a sign that weak ventricular contractions are not reaching the peripheral organs. If the pulse deficit is greater than 10, bring it to the doctor's attention. It could indicate atrial fibrillation or atrial or ventricular bigeminy. Remember either an increase or decrease in rate could be a sign of a cardiac disorder. For example, tachycardia is a sign of possible procainamide toxicity; bradycardia, a sign of propranolol and digitalis toxicity.

• *Heart rhythm:* Simultaneously, note heart rhythm and describe it in your notes. Also, describe the rhythm as the patient perceives it; some patients are able to beat out the rhythm they feel.

• *Blood pressure:* Measure every cardiac patient's blood pressure at least twice a day, oftener if you notice other abnormalities. Initially, take the blood pressure in both arms. Remember that, for every antiarrhythmic drug, hypotension is a sign of possible toxicity.

Being ready
To sum up, a key to good nursing for cardiac patients is to anticipate arrhythmias and to look for signs of them. Once you suspect an arrhythmia, do what the alert nurse did at the beginning of this chapter. Try to determine what drugs and equipment the doctor will need to treat the patient and have them ready.

What were the doctor's needs in Mr. Wiedman's case? Antiarrhythmic drugs, propranolol and lidocaine. Also D_5W, I.V. equipment, and a portable EKG. Because the nurse knew her drugs — and the patient's condition — she was able to act swiftly and decisively. Mr. Wiedman's arrhythmia was corrected and he was eventually discharged without further complications. Would this be true if he had been in your care?

SKILLCHECK 2

1. George Nicholson, a feeble 78-year-old, is admitted to the hospital with acute congestive heart failure. His medical history reveals that he has cirrhosis and hypothyroidism. The hypothyroidism has been controlled with sodium levothyroxine. Now the doctor plans to digitalize Mr. Nicholson and give him furosemide to relieve the edema from congestive heart failure. What should you watch for?

2. A 49-year-old train conductor, Albert Burke, is one week out of CCU where he was treated for atrial fibrillation. Now he's spiking temperatures of 101° F. (38.3° C.) and 102° F. (38.9° C.), though he shows no other signs of infection. He has a headache, and is weak, dizzy, and nauseated. Currently, he's taking the following oral drugs: digoxin, furosemide, and quinidine. What's causing Mr. Burke's symptoms?

3. Francis Lloyd is an 81-year-old retired carpenter who weighs only 115 pounds. He has been in the CCU for three days, after suffering an inferior wall MI. His recovery has been uncomplicated, and tests indicate that his heart damage is slight. The doctor hopes to digitalize Mr. Lloyd on digoxin over a period of three days. Without questioning the route of administration, the nurse gives the digoxin I.V. as she is accustomed to doing. Mr. Lloyd's heart rate, which had been between 80 and 90 beats per minute, slows and stabilizes at 64 beats per minute. He complains of headache and dizziness. What is wrong?

4. At 72, Mrs. Charity Wade still works as a cleaning woman. She's admitted to CCU with dyspnea, pitting edema of her ankles and shortness of breath on slight exertion. Chest X-ray confirms a diagnosis of congestive heart failure. She is digitalized and placed on a daily regime of digoxin, furosemide, and potassium chloride with a low salt diet. She is discharged on these drugs and given diet instructions.
   Two months later, Mrs. Wade goes to the clinic for a check-up. Ankle edema is noticeable. She tells you the swelling began yesterday but will go down soon because she took her water pill today. Questioning reveals that she takes her diuretic only when her ankles swell. What can you do to help Mrs. Wade?

5. Pat Lafferty, a 55-year-old bartender, has just been switched from I.V. lidocaine to oral procainamide to suppress premature extrasystoles. His doctor has also ordered chorothiazide because he's heard fine rales in Mr. Lafferty's left lung. Naturally, you've been watching the EKG monitor closely for any changes in the patient's heart rhythm and checking his blood pressure. Now you're alarmed, because Mr. Lafferty's blood pressure has dropped. Within 12 hours, it's gone from 120/78 to 106/60. Do you know why?

6. James Spears is a 45-year-old newspaper reporter who was just transferred to your unit from the CCU. One week earlier, he had an acute MI with moderate congestive heart failure. In the CCU, his congestive heart failure cleared up with digoxin and ethacrynic acid daily. Suddenly, he complains of skipped beats. Do you know what the doctor will suggest?

7. At 39, Joe Alexander was the youngest patient in the CCU. Earlier in the day, he was admitted with severe chest pain and his EKG showed signs of acute myocardial infarction. This evening, Mr. Alexander's heart rhythm changes from normal sinus to sinus bradycardia and PVCs begin occurring with increased frequency. On doctor's orders, you give Mr. Alexander lidocaine I.V. bolus and start a lidocaine I.V. drip at 60 microdrops/minute (4 mg) to suppress the ectopic ventricular beats. Two hours later, he complains that he feels cold, dizzy, and is nauseated. What's wrong?

8. Melvin Potter, a 50-year-old mechanic who weighs 230 pounds, is admitted to CCU from the emergency room with a tentative diagnosis of antero-lateral infarction. His temperature is normal, his blood pressure is 220/140, his pulse rate 68, and his respirations 22. When you question Mr. Potter, you learn that he has a long history of angina pectoris and for several months has been taking 20 mg propranolol four times a day to relieve pain.
   Now he tells you that he missed his first two doses of propranolol that day and has just taken his 4 o'clock dose. He has a "pounding headache" and substernal pain radiating into his left neck and jaw.
   You give Mr. Potter nitroprusside as ordered in an I.V. drip of D₅W, also I.M. morphine. His blood pressure lowers quickly, but his pulse also decreases to 58/min. Two hours later, you hear definite rales bilaterally in both lower chest lobes. Mr. Potter's respirations increase to 30/min and he says he is uncomfortable. You page the cardiologist. What might be the problem?

(Answers on page 166)

THE PREVENTIVE AGENTS

What are they? Antihypertensives…
anticoagulants and
antilipemics. What's your
role in administering them?
Gaining patient cooperation.

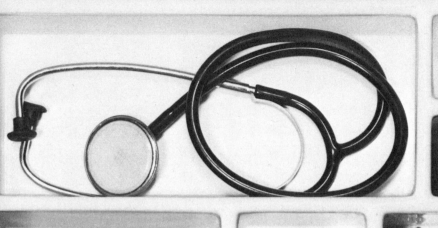
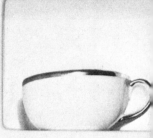
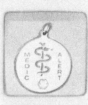
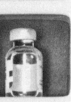
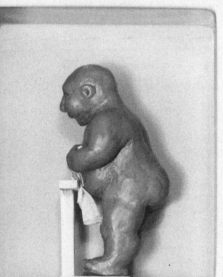
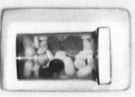
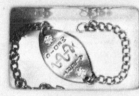
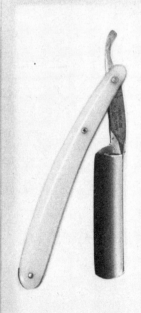

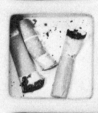
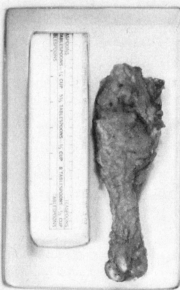
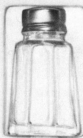
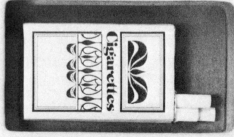
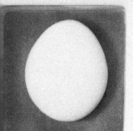
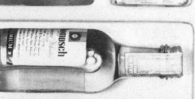
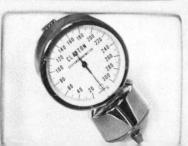

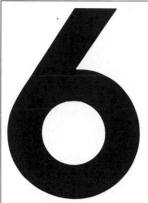

ANTIHYPERTENSIVES:
Gaining
patient cooperation

BY DANIEL A. HUSSAR, PhD

"I DON'T HAVE ANYTHING WRONG with me that a few days' vacation won't cure," grumbled Mr. Barnes, a 55-year-old newspaperman. But the nurse checked his blood pressure again anyway; it was 164/110.

Mr. Barnes had been admitted to the hospital for minor elective surgery, but it was postponed because of his moderate hypertension. Like many other patients, Mr. Barnes never suspected he had high blood pressure. He felt fine, and — except for being overweight — looked normal.

Is that unusual for hypertensive patients? Are most diaphoretic, edematous, weak or pale? Do they complain of palpitations, nausea, diarrhea, or dizziness? Some hypertensive patients have these signs and symptoms, but most — like Mr. Barnes — do not. They're asymptomatic. That's why they're difficult to diagnose and care for. Without a sphygmomanometer handy, neither you nor patients may suspect high blood pressure.

Hypertensive emergencies, of course, are the exception. They make patients gravely ill, requiring constant attention with appropriate drugs in the emergency room or CCU (see Chapter 10). Walking hypertensives, by comparison, may not even consider themselves sick. This creates special problems for you and everyone else caring for them.

For example, many hypertensive patients don't take the drugs they're given as ordered. Why? Because they complain that their drug's side effects are worse than the disease. Little wonder, then, that most of them aren't even close to optimal control. The doctor is treating a disease that — until complications occur — remains asymptomatic. And he's doing it with drugs that produce disagreeable or even dangerous side effects.

The key to gaining patient cooperation under these circumstances is patient education. Each patient must be told why his hypertension is dangerous and why he must follow doctor's orders. As you know, even mild hypertension is progressive, leading to accelerated atherosclerosis, renal dysfunction, and ultimately death. The prognosis for *untreated* hypertension depends on its severity. The higher the diastolic pressure, the higher the morbidity and mortality.

As a nurse, you'll be partly responsible for teaching the patient about his disease. And you must do it in a way that he can understand and adapt to. To achieve this, you'll need to know a lot about antihypertensive drugs — how they work and why certain ones are chosen. What, for example, are their side effects? How do they interact with other drugs? And how are they affected by physiological and environmental factors? All this information is important, so that you can care for your patient properly.

Who needs treatment?
Most doctors use these guidelines to decide which hypertensive patients need treatment:

• The need for treatment is absolute and may be urgent if diastolic pressure exceeds 130 mm Hg, especially if one of the following complications exists: hypertensive encephalopathy or cerebrovascular accident, retinal hemorrhage, congestive heart failure, acute nephritis, preeclampsia, or renal azotemia. With these conditions, many patients require hospitalization for treatment with potent antihypertensives; the patients will be discharged only when their blood pressure is well controlled and when they're thoroughly indoctrinated in long-term therapy (see Chapter 10).

• Treatment with antihypertensive drugs should also be ini-

NURSES' GUIDE TO
COMMON ANTIHYPERTENSIVES

GENERIC NAME	TRADE NAME	ROUTE AND DOSAGE	COMMON SIDE EFFECTS
Antiadrenergic drugs: Rauwolfia alkaloids			
whole root rauwolfia	Rauwolfia Raudixin◇	P.O.: 50-400 mg daily, in divided doses taken a.m. and p.m.	Depression, GI disturbances, angina-like symptoms, arrhythmias, drowsiness, nervousness, anxiety, nightmares, dull sensorium, deafness, nasal congestion, pruritus, rash, dry mouth, dizziness, headache, impotence, dysuria, muscular aches, weight gain, fluid retention, loss of appetite
alseroxylon	Rautensin Rauwiloid	P.O.: Initial dose 2-4 mg daily. Maintenance 2 mg daily	
reserpine	Reserpine Reserpanca◇◇ Neo-serp◇◇ Serpasil◇	P.O.: Initial dose 0.5 mg daily for 1-2 weeks. Maintenance 0.1-0.25 mg daily. I.M. (hypertensive crisis): Initial dose 0.5-1.0 mg, then 2-4 mg q3h until desired response	
deserpidine	Harmonyl	P.O.: Initial dose 0.75-1.0 mg daily for 10-14 days, when full response is apparent. Maintenance 0.25 mg daily	
rescinnamine	Moderil	P.O.: 0.25-0.5 mg daily	
syrosingopine	Singoserp	P.O.: 0.5-3 mg daily	
Other antiadrenergics			
methyldopa	Aldomet◇	P.O.: Initial dose 250 mg 2-3 times daily for 2 days, then increase or decrease dose every 2 days until desired effect obtained. Maintenance 500 mg-2 G daily in 2-4 doses I.V. infusion: 100 mg-3 G in 100 ml 5% glucose in water over 30-60 minutes q6h (dose titrated according to blood pressure)	Orthostatic hypotension, transient sedation, headache, weakness, dizziness, light-headedness, nightmares, depression, bradycardia, anginal pain, edema, dry mouth, sore tongue, rash, nasal stuffiness, gynecomastia, impotence, decreased libido, arthralgia, myalgia

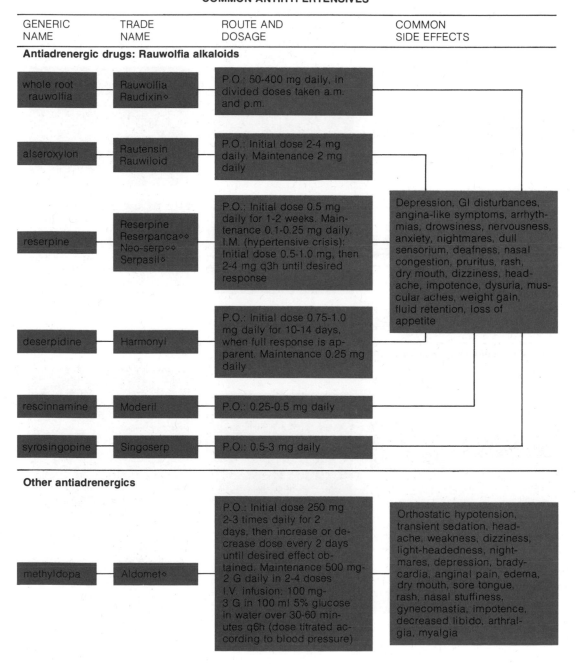

NURSES' GUIDE TO
COMMON ANTIHYPERTENSIVES

GENERIC NAME	TRADE NAME	ROUTE AND DOSAGE	COMMON SIDE EFFECTS
Other antiadrenergics (continued)			
guanethidine sulfate	Ismelin◊	P.O.: 25-50 mg daily	Orthostatic hypotension, dizziness, weakness, lassitude, syncope, bradycardia, dyspnea, GI disturbance, dry mouth, ptosis, blurred vision, angina, muscle tremor, nasal congestion, asthma, diarrhea, impotence, fluid retention
clonidine hydrochloride	Catapres	P.O.: Initial dose 0.1 mg b.i.d. Maintenance increase by 0.1-0.2 mg per day until desired response obtained; usual range is 0.2-0.8 mg daily in divided doses	Dry mouth, drowsiness, sedation, dizziness, headache, fatigue, GI disturbances, insomnia, depression, rash, urticaria, urinary retention, impotence, fluid retention
propranolol (See antiarrhythmic chart)			
Vascular smooth-muscle relaxants			
hydralazine	Hydralazine Apresoline◊ Lopress	P.O.: Initial dose 10 mg q.i.d. for 4 days, then 25 mg q.i.d. for 3 days, then 50 mg q.i.d. thereafter. Maintenance lowest effective dose I.V., I.M.: 20-40 mg repeated as necessary	Orthostatic hypotension, headache, palpitations, GI disturbance, tachycardia, angina, nasal congestion, flushing, lacrimation, conjunctivitis, paresthesia, numbness, tingling, edema, dizziness, tremors, muscle cramps, depression, disorientation, anxiety, rash, urinary difficulty, dyspnea, paralytic ileus
prazosin hydrochloride	Minipress	P.O.: Initial dose 1 mg t.i.d. Maintenance 20-40 mg daily in divided doses	Severe syncope with loss of consciousness if initial dose greater than 1 mg, headache, drowsiness, weakness, palpitations, GI disturbance, edema, dyspnea, tachycardia, depression, nervousness, paresthesia, rash, blurred vision, tinnitus, dry mouth, diaphoresis

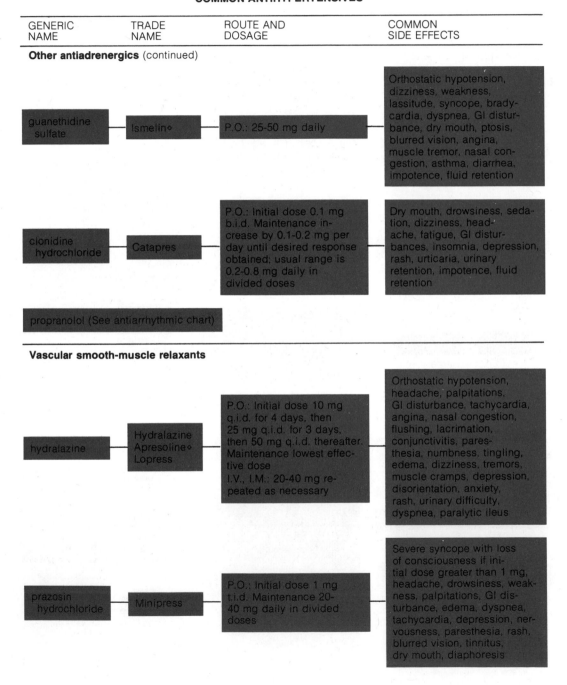

NURSES' GUIDE TO
COMMON ANTIHYPERTENSIVES

GENERIC NAME	TRADE NAME	ROUTE AND DOSAGE	COMMON SIDE EFFECTS
Vascular smooth-muscle relaxants			
nitroprusside sodium	Nipride◇	I.V. infusion: 50 mg/250-1000 ml 5% glucose in water infused at 0.5-10 mcg/Kg/min (smaller dose used for patients receiving concomitant antihypertensive medications)	GI disturbance, increased perspiration, headache, restlessness, apprehension, muscle twitching, retrosternal discomfort, palpitations, dizziness, irritation at infusion site
diazoxide	Hyperstat◇◇	I.V.: 300 mg rapidly I.V. push (slow injection may fail to reduce blood pressure), repeat in ½ hour if required, then q4-24h for 4-5 days	Angina, arrhythmias, cerebral ischemia, rash, fever, increased perspiration, flushing, palpitations, bradycardia, headache, dizziness, light-headedness, tinnitus, momentary hearing loss, weakness
tolazine hydrochloride (also adrenergic blocker)	Priscoline	P.O.: Initial dose 25 mg q4-6h p.c. Dosage gradually increased to desired level. I.V., I.M., S.C., 25-75 mg q.i.d.	Flushing, sensation of chilliness or warmth at beginning of therapy, tachycardia, tingling, nausea, and epigastric distress, postural hypotension
Ganglionic blocking agents			
mecamylamine hydrochloride	Inversine	P.O.: Initial dose 2.5 mg b.i.d., increase by increments of 2.5 mg every 2 days until desired effect attained. Maintenance 2.5-25 mg daily in divided doses	Anorexia, dry mouth, nausea, vomiting, constipation, paralytic ileus, weakness, fatigue, sedation, orthostatic, syncope paresthesia, blurred vision, dilated pupils, urinary retention, pulmonary edema
trimethaphan camsylate	Arfonad	I.V. infusion: 10 ml/500 ml 5% glucose in water, start at 3-4 mg/min; regulate dosage according to blood pressure readings	Severe hypotension, dilated pupils, respiratory depression, tachycardia

For other common antihypertensive drugs and their dosages, see Appendices.

tiated in patients with diastolic pressures between 110 and 130 mm Hg, even in the absence of complications (e.g., cardiovascular or renal manifestations).

• Treatment is indicated for most patients with diastolic pressures between 95 and 110 mm Hg, and with complications such as headaches, or cardiovascular or renal manifestations. Even without complications, diuretic or other therapy is justified.

Doctors must weigh several other factors before deciding which drugs to use:

• Age: Elevated blood pressure in young people is more dangerous than in the old.

• Concomitant disease: Diseases that decrease kidney function may make patients more sensitive to antihypertensive drugs.

• Sex: The risk of stroke or heart attack from sustained hypertension is greater in men than women; hence, therapy is more urgent for men.

• Race: Black people develop hypertension earlier; it's more severe, with a higher mortality at a younger age.

• Occupation: If the patient's occupation requires high mental and physical alertness, using a drug such as reserpine may be undesirable.

• Emotional status: Depressed patients should not receive reserpine or its analogs.

How the drugs work
Many antihypertensive drugs are available, but you can divide the ones used most into three main groups:

• Diuretics
• Drugs that inhibit the sympathetic system
• Drugs that act on the vascular smooth muscle.

All these work directly or indirectly to reduce peripheral vascular resistance, decreasing the heart's workload and lowering blood pressure. For most patients, doctors combine them. This enhances the good effects of each drug and — by reducing dosages — minimizes the bad.

Diuretics, unless specifically contraindicated, are chosen first to treat patients with mild-to-moderate hypertension. Chapter 3 explains how — in some cases — they lower blood pressure without the addition of other antihypertensive drugs.

Drugs that inhibit the patient's sympathetic nervous system

HOW ANTIHYPERTENSIVES ACT ON THE AUTONOMIC NERVOUS SYSTEM

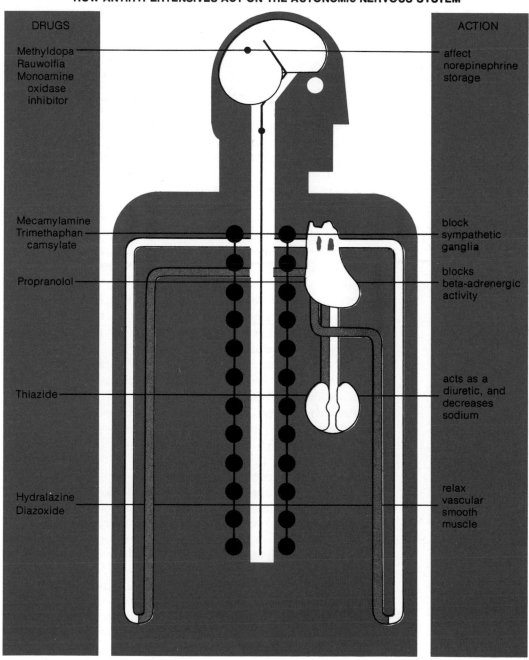

DRUGS

Methyldopa
Rauwolfia
Monoamine
 oxidase
 inhibitor

Mecamylamine
Trimethaphan
 camsylate

Propranolol

Thiazide

Hydralazine
Diazoxide

ACTION

affect
norepinephrine
storage

block
sympathetic
ganglia

blocks
beta-adrenergic
activity

acts as a
diuretic, and
decreases
sodium

relax
vascular
smooth
muscle

are subdivided into two types: those that block transmission of only sympathetic nerve impulses (antiadrenergic drugs); and those that block transmission of both sympathetic and parasympathetic nerve impulses at the ganglia (ganglionic-blocking drugs). For a detailed explanation of the cardiovascular and autonomic nervous system, see Chapter 1.

Of the two types, ganglionic-blocking drugs (for example, trimethaphan camsylate) are used mostly for hypertensive emergencies, because they act rapidly and dissipate quickly (see Chapter 10).

Antiadrenergic drugs include the rauwolfia preparations (of which reserpine is the prototype) as well as methyldopa, guanethidine, and propranolol.

Reserpine

Reserpine is almost always used with other antihypertensive drugs for patients with mild-to-moderate hypertension. It acts as a tranquilizer, as well as a hypotensive, benefitting the patient whose hypertension is aggravated by tension and anxiety. Because it dissipates slowly, reserpine keeps a patient's blood pressure from rising suddenly if he accidentally misses a dose. This makes it particularly useful for patients who are elderly or forgetful.

Despite these benefits, many doctors prefer other antihypertensive drugs instead of reserpine. The reason: reserpine's high incidence of undesirable side effects, the most dangerous of which is severe mental depression. Watch any patient on reserpine for signs of depression — it usually comes on gradually, but may lead the patient to suicide if it becomes severe. Notify the doctor immediately if the patient seems despondent or complains of nightmares, early morning insomnia, or loss of appetite. He will discontinue the drug.

Nasal stuffiness and dryness of the mouth are two of reserpine's least serious side effects. But they may be troublesome to your patient, so call them to the doctor's attention.

Other possible side effects include nausea, vomiting, diarrhea, abdominal cramps, drowsiness, fluid retention, angina-like symptoms, arrhythmias (particularly when used with other drugs), and bradycardia. Bradycardia, however, may be desirable, as in hypertensive patients with tachycardia or those receiving hydralazine, which can cause tachycardia. The doctor will probably give the patient a diuretic to relieve fluid retention, which could cause edema.

Reserpine is not given to pregnant or lactating women, because it crosses the placental barrier and is secreted in breast milk.

Methyldopa

Another drug, methyldopa, has fewer side effects than reserpine and works well in patients with moderate hypertension. It's used for many patients with impaired kidney function, because it doesn't significantly affect renal blood flow. (Some doctors, however, prefer hydralazine for such patients.)

Methyldopa is seldom used by itself because its antihypertensive effect is erratic, and the patient develops a tolerance to it usually within 2 to 3 months. It's generally more effective combined with a diuretic.

The patient is more likely to suffer orthostatic hypotension with methyldopa than with reserpine, hydralazine, or diuretics. But the risk is less than with guanethidine or the ganglionic-blocking drugs. Thus methyldopa may be useful in treating patients with cerebrovascular or coronary insufficiency, which may be aggravated by sudden orthostatic decreases in blood pressure.

Almost half the patients on methyldopa experience drowsiness, but it generally diminishes as their treatment continues. Salt and water retention occurs, but can be relieved with diuretics. Other possible side effects include dryness of the mouth, gastrointestinal upsets, diarrhea, nasal stuffiness, fever, nightmares, and loss of libido.

In a patient who has been on methyldopa for 6 months or more, watch for a positive reaction to a direct Coombs' test. It may mean he's developing hemolytic anemia from the drug, although only a small percentage (0.1% - 0.2%) of patients with a positive reaction do. In rare cases, the patient's urine may darken on exposure to air, because of the breakdown of methyldopa.

Guanethidine

Guanethidine is still another drug that inhibits the sympathetic nervous system. It's a potent adrenergic blocker, which many doctors prefer — in combination with other drugs — for severe hypertension. Yet, it's also for patients with mild-to-moderate hypertension who don't respond to other antihypertensives.

DRUG INTERACTIONS — ANTIHYPERTENSIVES

THIS DRUG	TAKEN WITH	INTERACTION
guanethidine	alcohol	Causes orthostatic hypotension and drowsiness
	amphetamine	Inhibits guanethidine effects
	antidepressant (tricyclic)	Inhibits guanethidine effects
	doxepin	Decreases antihypertensive effect
	ephedrine	Decreases antihypertensive effect
	levarterenol (norepinephrine)	Increases antihypertensive effect, cardiac arrhythmias
	methylphenidate	Decreases antihypertensive effect
	MAO inhibitor	Decreases antihypertensive effect
	phenothiazine especially chlorpromazine	Antagonizes guanethidine
	phenylephrine	Increases phenylephrine effects; increases pupillary response with eye drops
	metaraminol	Increases antihypertensive effects; decreases vasopressor effects
methyldopa	amphetamine	Decreases antihypertensive effect
	anesthetic	Causes hypotension
	propranolol	Increases antihypertensive effects

DRUG INTERACTIONS — ANTIHYPERTENSIVES

THIS DRUG	TAKEN WITH	INTERACTION
methyldopa	sympathomimetic	Decreases antihypertensive effects
	methotrimeprazine	Causes orthostatic hypotension
pargyline	alcohol	Decreases MAO inhibitor; causes hypertensive crisis
	amphetamine	Increases amphetamine effects
	barbiturate	Increases barbiturate effects
	food containing tyramine	Decreases MAO inhibitor; causes hypertensive crisis
	insulin	Increases insulin effects
	levodopa	Increases levodopa effects
	methyldopa	Causes excitation and hypertension
	reserpine	Causes excitation and hypertension
	sympathomimetic	Increases sympathomimetic effect
	tricyclic antidepressant	Increases antidepressant effects; causes hyperpyrexia, convulsions
reserpine	digitalis	Induces cardiac arrhythmias
	MAO inhibitor	Causes excitation and hypertension
	ephedrine	Decreases ephedrine effect

Guanethidine also benefits patients with renal hypertension when it's used with a diuretic.

Guanethidine produces many side effects, however. Orthostatic hypotension is one of the worst and occurs in many patients. It's usually most marked in the morning, so warn your patient not to get out of bed too quickly. Also tell him to avoid heavy exercise, alcohol, and hot weather. Advise him to sit or lie down immediately if he feels weak or dizzy.

Patients on guanethidine may complain about diarrhea after meals. They may also experience impotence, nausea, fatigue, fluid retention, muscle tremor, nasal stuffiness, dry mouth or blurred vision.

One thing in guanethidine's favor: It doesn't cross the blood-brain barrier, so it's not apt to cause depression like reserpine.

Propranolol

Propranolol is a beta adrenergic blocker that's used in combination with other drugs to treat almost every degree of hypertension. About the only contraindications are asthma, congestive heart failure, or second- or third-degree heart block. The danger here: Propranolol lowers the heart rate and diminishes myocardial contractility.

This drug must also be used with caution in diabetics, because its action may prevent tachycardia and tremor that serve as signs of insulin-induced hypoglycemia.

Many doctors find it particularly useful with hydralazine, because it blocks some of hydralazine's adverse side effects; for example, reflex tachycardia.

Most hypertensive patients accept propranolol well, because it has few disagreeable side effects. It causes little or no impotence, as reserpine and methyldopa do; it doesn't cause orthostatic hypotension or dry mouth. However, some patients complain of fatigue, lethargy, or gastrointestinal discomfort from it. A few have other side effects: skin rash, reversible alopecia or hallucinations.

Propranolol is also used effectively for patients with angina pectoris and certain arrhythmias. (See Chapters 4 and 5.)

Clonidine

One of the newest antihypertensive drugs is clonidine. Like other antiadrenergic drugs, it inhibits the sympathetic nervous

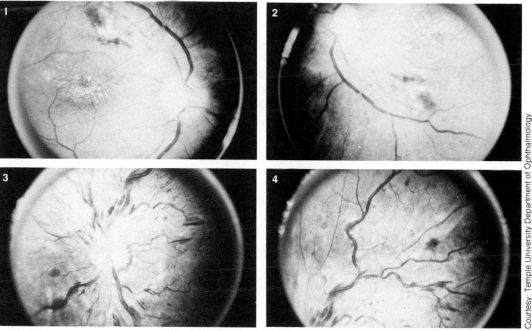

Courtesy: Temple University Department of Ophthalmology

system, but it does so by affecting the central nervous system. It slows the heart rate, decreasing cardiac output. This, in turn, reduces peripheral vascular resistance and lowers the patient's blood pressure. Doctors use clonidine in combination with other drugs to treat mild-to-moderate hypertension.

The most important thing to teach the patient about clonidine is to take the drug as ordered. If he discontinues it abruptly, his blood pressure may rise rapidly. He may also have nervousness, tremor, headache, nausea, or increased salivation. These symptoms begin to appear a few hours after a dose is missed.

Taking the drug on schedule, however, he may have other side effects. For example, constipation, dry mouth, drowsiness, dizziness, or fluid retention. Clonidine may also increase depression and, possibly, cause degenerative retinal changes. Urge patients taking this drug to have their eyes examined periodically by an ophthalmologist.

Vascular smooth-muscle relaxants: hydralazine and prazosin
Of the drugs that act on the vascular smooth muscle, hydralazine is usually favored for treating mild-to-moderate

The eyes have it
These photos show some of the degenerative retinal changes patients with hypertension may suffer. Figures 1 and 2 are the eye grounds of a 40-year-old man. Although he had no visual complaints, his blood pressure on admission was 250/150.

Figures 3 and 4 are the eye grounds of a 43-year-old woman. She had malignant hypertension, blurred vision, papilledema of the left disc, fresh hemorrhage, and impending vein occlusion.

All of these fundus photos are classified as Grade III changes.

hypertension. Even so, it's usually reserved for use as a third drug when a two-drug combination is ineffective.

Hydralazine has two advantages: It doesn't make the patient drowsy, nor significantly decrease renal blood flow. The latter advantage makes it particularly useful for patients with impaired renal function, such as those with preeclampsia or acute glomerulonephritis.

Because hydralazine produces so many adverse side effects, doctors usually combine it with other drugs so they can reduce its dosage. Possible side effects include orthostatic hypotension, headache, palpitations, anorexia, nausea, vomiting, diarrhea, and tachycardia. A syndrome known as "hydralazine disease" develops in about 10% of patients taking more than 200 mg daily over a prolonged period. The syndrome resembles acute rheumatoid arthritis, and even a lupus erythematosus-like ailment if the drug is not promptly discontinued.

Prazosin is a smooth-muscle relaxant similar to hydralazine. It produces fewer side effects, but may cause dizziness followed by loss of consciousness 30 to 90 minutes after first dose (unless it's no more than 1 mg). This is called a "first-dose phenomenon."

Dizziness may also occur if the doctor increases the dose too rapidly or adds another antihypertensive drug. Watch the patient closely and warn him to call his doctor if he has dizziness.

Why some patients are uncooperative

As I said earlier in this chapter, side effects from antihypertensives may seem worse than the disease to many patients. This was the case with Mr. Barnes, the newspaperman whose hypertension was discovered during a preoperative blood pressure check.

During his hospital stay, Mr. Barnes' hypertension was regulated with hydrochlorothiazide, 50 mg once daily, and methyldopa, 250 mg four times daily. When he was discharged, his blood pressure was 130/80. He was told to keep his salt intake down and report for a checkup in 1 month.

After discharge, Mr. Barnes resumed work and all his former activities. He complained to his wife that he felt drowsy and lethargic, but otherwise well. During the second week after discharge, he felt so well he eased up on his diet,

Dear Patient:
Here's what you should know about the drug your doctor has prescribed for you.
Methyldopa is used to treat high blood pressure. It will bring your blood pressure into a normal range and help keep it there.

To make sure you get the most from your therapy, follow these instructions carefully:

1. Take methyldopa only as prescribed. Never skip a dose or increase, decrease, or change your dose in any way without an order from your doctor.
2. Stay on the diet your doctor has given you. Don't drink alcohol without asking him first.
3. Tell every doctor who treats you that you are taking methyldopa.
4. Because methyldopa can cause drowsiness, be careful if you have to drive or perform other tasks that require mental alertness. This drowsiness usually disappears with time.
5. Avoid sudden rising or prolonged standing. If you have been lying down or sitting for a long period of time, stand up slowly to avoid dizziness.

Call the doctor *immediately* if you notice any of the following: depression, dizziness, fainting, mouth dryness, extreme drowsiness, nasal congestion, fatigue, headache, numbness, constipation, fever, rash, joint pains, impotence, nightmares, confusion, dark urine, excessive bruising, or changes in skin color.

Dear Patient:
Here's what you should know about the drug your doctor has prescribed for you.
Reserpine is used to treat high blood pressure. It will bring your blood pressure into a normal range and help keep it there.

To make sure you get the most from your therapy, follow these instructions carefully:

1. Take this drug only as prescribed. Never skip a dose, increase it, or decrease it without asking your doctor.
2. Stay on the diet your doctor has given you.
3. Tell every doctor who treats you that you are taking this drug, especially if he plans surgery or you will be given an anesthetic.
4. This drug can cause drowsiness (which will disappear in time). Be careful if you have to drive or perform other tasks that require mental alertness.
5. Avoid sudden rising or prolonged standing. Stand up slowly to avoid dizziness.
6. *Notify your doctor if you become pregnant.*

Call the doctor immediately if you notice any of the following: depression, dizziness, fainting, diarrhea, stomach distress, black stools, weight gain greater than 2 lbs in 1 day or 7 lbs in 1 week, chest pains, heart palpitations, impotence, nightmares, rash, nasal congestion, or hives.

occasionally forgot to take his pills, and soon discontinued them entirely. Feeling much better, he supposed his high blood pressure had been due to increased tension he experienced going to the hospital for elective surgery. He didn't return to the doctor for a checkup.

Six weeks after discharge, however, Mr. Barnes returned to the hospital for the minor elective surgery. The admitting nurse noted that he had gained 3 pounds since discharge, then checked his blood pressure. It was 180/120. Mr. Barnes was incredulous. "There must be a mistake," he gasped. Like many other patients who discontinue antihypertensive drugs and feel better, Mr. Barnes thought his blood pressure was now normal.

This time, Mr. Barnes got a lot more instruction from both doctor and nurses before he was discharged. And that's the key to gaining cooperation from any patient on antihypertensive drugs — adequate teaching.

Teaching the patient what to expect

Using the examples on page 103 as a guide, make up a card that will teach the patient everything he should know about his disease and therapy. Include the specific side effects he may experience with the drugs he's taking. (As you can see, patient teaching cards for methyldopa and reserpine are included in this chapter. You will find cards for guanethidine and clonidine in Chapter 10.) Warn him never to alter the dosage of his drugs in any way or add nonprescription drugs without specific instructions from his doctor.

By properly teaching the patient about antihypertensives, you'll increase the chances of his staying on these necessary drugs. You may also encourage him to endure the side effects caused by many of these drugs. And you'll certainly improve his health, which is what good nursing is all about.

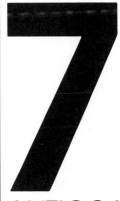

ANTICOAGULANTS: Teaching the do's and don'ts

BY DANIEL A. HUSSAR, PhD

GIVING ANTICOAGULANT DRUGS imposes a great responsibility on you — more responsibility than other cardiac drugs, even digitalis. But nobody needs to tell you that, especially with the extraordinary precautions many hospitals take. Several hospitals, for example, require that all charts be initialed by *two* nurses, certifying that the lab report of clotting time is in hand and that the syringe has been double-checked, before heparin can be administered.

Extraordinary precautions, yes. But they make sense. When a doctor orders anticoagulant therapy, he deliberately upsets a delicate balance between the factors in the blood that promote clot formation and those that *inhibit* it. He deliberately pushes the patient to the brink of hemorrhage. He gambles: accepting a risk of hemorrhage in the hopes of reducing the more lethal risk of thromboembolism.

The difficulty is this: Since patients' reactions to anticoagulants are individualized, their treatment must be individualized, too. Anticoagulant effects must be followed closely with repeated laboratory tests; you must watch the patient carefully for any tendency toward hemorrhage.

Your main job is proper patient education — providing

enough information to protect your patient from danger without frightening him so much he stops his therapy altogether. This chapter will give you tips for doing that.

How anticoagulants work

Anticoagulant therapy prevents enlargement of an existing thrombus (which might block the vascular channel) and formation of new thrombi. Two *main* types of anticoagulant drugs have long been used:

• *Heparin,* a parenteral anticoagulant that prevents clot extension directly by retarding the formation of fibrin, thereby prolonging the blood clotting time.

• *Warfarin,* an oral anticoagulant derivative of coumarin. It acts in the liver to inhibit vitamin K in the production of prothrombin and several other clotting factors. The oral anticoagulants act indirectly, leaving active clotting factors circulating in the blood. These drugs act slowly, as compared to heparin, since the body's supply of prothrombin and several other clotting factors must first be exhausted before the clotting time changes. Their effects last several days after the drugs get discontinued.

Heparin has been called the body's natural anticoagulant because it's found in the liver (which explains the origin of its name), in the lungs, and in the spleen. It reduces blood lipid levels, which may also benefit coronary patients, although the value of this has not yet been established.

Heparin is usually given intravenously, either intermittently or continuously. The most common method of administration is the I.V. intermittent bolus injection. Since heparin has a short half-life — around 60 minutes or so — never give bolus doses more often than every 4 hours. To check the effectiveness of heparin, have blood drawn for lab tests one-half hour before the next dose is due. This level should always be therapeutic. If not, dosage adjustment is necessary.

Some doctors prefer continuous infusion, however. It has 8-10 times lower incidence of major bleeding than bolus injections. Continuous infusion has disadvantages, too. It needs close monitoring of the administration. Use an I.V. pump or controller to lessen the risk of inadvertent overdoses caused by too fast an infusion. Or, use a 100 ml burette chamber and fill it hourly.

Because a single I.V. injection lasts only about 4 hours,

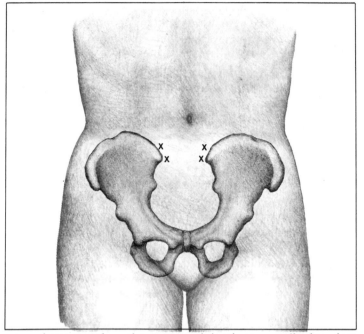

Injection tips
So they won't develop ecchymoses, teach patients using subcutaneous heparin to rotate the injection sites along the abdominal fat pad above the iliac crest. Make sure patients don't rub the site with an alcohol sponge, as this increases the absorption time. Instead, after an injection have the patient merely hold the sponge on the site for a few seconds.

some doctors order subcutaneous injections, usually deep into the abdominal fat pad or lateral thigh. This route provides longer drug action, but the absorption may be unpredictable and erratic, and the patient risks local hematomas. Occasionally, however, the doctor will place a patient leaving the hospital on subcutaneous heparin. Before he is released, teach the patient how to draw up the correct dose into a syringe. Then have him practice giving injections on an orange until he gains confidence. Teach him to rotate the injection sites on his lower abdomen so that his skin does not harden and develop ecchymoses. The I.M. route is not used because of tissue irritation.

To insure accuracy, all heparin doses are stated in units because the milligram potency of the available products is not uniform. Dosage depends on the patient's age, sex, and body surface area; the route of administration; any concurrent drug therapy; and the blood clotting time, which should be 2½ to 3 times the normal control, when the Lee-White whole blood clotting time method is used. The APTT test is an alternate screening test; therapeutic levels are twice the normal control of 35 to 45 seconds. Be careful with patients who may have pulmonary embolism; it may decrease the heparin's half-life.

To insure adequate anticoagulation, patients must receive their medication on time. Don't delay a heparin dose by waiting for blood to be drawn first. And unless a doctor orders you to, don't delay a scheduled dose by waiting for the lab results. If the lab technician isn't available to draw blood at the prescribed time, notify the doctor that heparin is due and blood hasn't been drawn. The doctor will tell you what to do. If you can't reach the doctor in 5 minutes, give the heparin on schedule anyway. Keep trying to reach him and inform him why the blood wasn't drawn. Only if a patient has nosebleeds, ecchymoses, bloody urine, or other side effects should you withhold a heparin dose. In that case, notify the doctor or your supervisor immediately.

Oral anticoagulants aren't used in acute cases, because they take 2 to 3 days to have an effect. However, they do have advantages over heparin. These advantages are:
- greater convenience for prolonged therapy
- uniform strength made possible by synthetic production
- less expense
- easier control of anticoagulation because of longer action.

To evaluate and control oral anticoagulants, doctors use the prothrombin time test. Based on control value, therapeutic range will be 2 to 2½ times control. Tests are needed daily until the maintenance dose is determined. Thereafter, many doctors feel a 2-week interval between tests will provide satisfactory control.

Because an anticoagulant's effectiveness is linked to clotting factors, you'll have to control your patient's vitamin K intake and fat intake to stabilize his response.

Several other phenomena affect patient response. Decreased liver or kidney function enhances response; diarrhea may reduce response by rushing the drugs through the gastrointestinal tract, reducing absorption. Because these things alter patient response unpredictably, you must be especially alert for evidence of bleeding tendencies.

Treatment for risk
Who needs anticoagulants? Anyone in danger of clot formation. This includes patients with the following disorders:
- *Thrombophlebitis*. This was the first disorder anticoagulants were given for, and the one they're most effective against.

GENERIC NAME	TRADE NAME	ROUTE AND DOSAGE	COMMON SIDE EFFECTS
heparin sodium	Heparin sodium Hepalean◇◇	Intermittent I.V.: Initially 10,000 units, then 5,000-10,000 units q4-6h Continuous I.V.: 20,000 to 40,000 units 1000 cc solution infused in 24-hour period (initial loading dose of 5,000 units should be given direct I.V. before continuous infusion) S.C.: Initially 10,000-20,000 units then 8,000-10,000 units q8h or 12,000-20,000 units q12h	GI bleeding (tarry stools, hematemesis), wound hematoma, hemarthrosis, adrenal hemorrhage with resultant acute renal insufficiency; hypersensitivity reaction most commonly manifested by chills, fever, urticaria, osteoporosis and suppression of renal function after long-term therapy; delayed transient alopecia; aldosterone suppression; rebound hyperlipemia following discontinuation
aspirin (acetylsalicylic acid)	Aspirin◇ A.S.A. (plain or time-released)	P.O.: 600 mg b.i.d.	Rapid and deep breathing, nausea, vomiting, vertigo, tinnitus, flushing, increased perspiration

Coumarin derivatives

dicumarol	Dicumarol Dufalone◇◇	P.O.: Initial day 200-300 mg then 25-200 mg on subsequent days if prothrombin activity is 25% or more of normal	Hemorrhage may occur though dose and prothrombin time in normal range; GI bleeding, hematuria, nephropathy, blood dyscrasias, rash, pruritus, urticaria, alopecia, fever, sore throat and mouth, petechiae, ecchymosis, bleeding from mucous membranes, wound hemorrhage, paralytic ileus, uterine bleeding, hemorrhagic necrosis of female breast, epistaxis, cerebral hemorrhage, fetal hemorrhage if given during pregnancy, prothrombinopenic state in infant if given to lactating mother
phenprocoumon	Liquamar Marcumar◇◇	P.O.: Induction 24 mg; maintenance 0.75-6.0 mg	
warfarin sodium	Coumadin sodium◇ Panwarfin Warfilone◇◇ Warnerim◇◇	P.O., I.M., I.V.: Initially 20-40 mg divided over a period of 2-4 days (average dose 10 mg); maintenance dose range 2-10 mg in accordance with protime determinations	
warfarin potassium	Anthrombin-K◇	P.O.: Initially 40-60 mg daily, then 2.5-10 mg daily	
acenocoumarol	Sintrom◇	P.O.: 16-28 mg first day, 8-16 mg second day, then daily maintenance 2-10 mg	

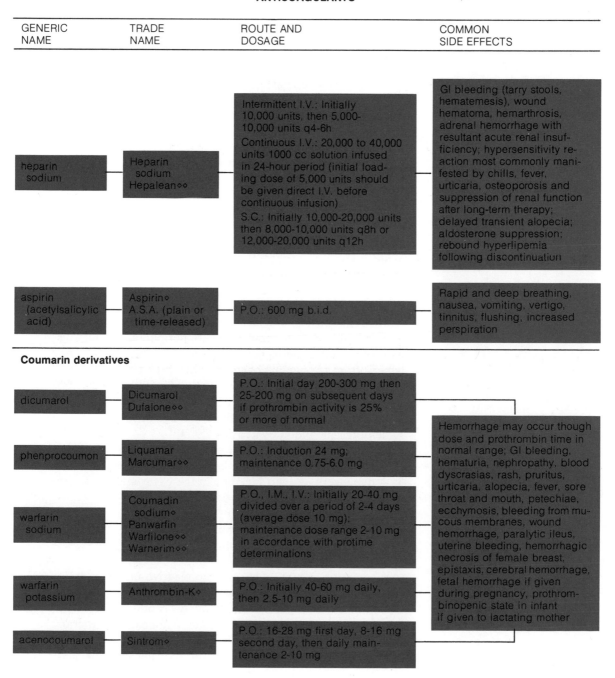

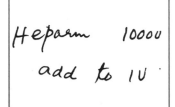

Heparin   10000

add to IU

A deathly mistake
Confusing abbreviations, such as
the one above, are responsible for
dangerous drug errors. Be sure
you write out the word units to
avoid giving your patients an
overdose.

• *Surgery, immobilization, or trauma.* Doctors give anti-coagulants to prevent blood clots after cardiac valve replacement; during long immobilization; after peripheral arterial embolization; after hip, pelvis, and femur fracture; for cerebrovascular disease accompanied by transient ischemic attack and for rheumatic heart disease.

• *Congestive heart failure.* About 50% of heart failure patients with chronic edema of the lower extremities develop pulmonary emboli, often without associated infarction. So, doctors recommend anticoagulants for patients with recurrent embolization. Some recommend it for all patients with persistent leg edema secondary to heart failure.

• *Myocardial infarction.* Giving anticoaglants for myocardial infarction is controversial because anticoagulants don't dissolve existing clots, nor can they prevent further infarction. Many doctors do prescribe them, however, for patients with acute infarction, especially those with previous infarction, congestive heart failure, arrhythmias, deep venous thrombosis, or pulmonary embolism. Although the benefit to such patients is not certain, they're not harmed if maintained within therapeutic range. Long-term therapy is generally not recommended, although men under 60 with peripheral vascular disease, who suffer the highest incidence of recurrent MI, may benefit from taking anticoagulants for up to 1 year.

Contraindications: When the risk is too great
Here are 7 contraindications for anticoagulant therapy:
1. hemorrhagic blood dyscrasias
2. recent or impending surgery of the central nervous system or eye, or surgery creating large open surfaces
3. active ulcers or overt bleeding in the gastrointestinal, genitourinary, or respiratory tract
4. cerebrovascular hemorrhage
5. aneurysms or increased capillary fragility
6. subacute bacterial endocarditis
7. threatened abortion.

When your patient must undergo elective minor or major surgery or tooth extraction, the doctor will probably want to discontinue anticoagulants and allow his prothrombin time to fall below 1½ times the control value. Anticoagulant therapy can be reinstituted after the procedure is over.

Certain other conditions *may* contraindicate anticoagulants

DRUG INTERACTIONS — ANTICOAGULANTS

THIS DRUG	TAKEN WITH	INTERACTION
bishydroxycoumarin or warfarin	aminosalicylic acid, salicylate	Increases anticoagulant effect
	barbiturate	Decreases anticoagulant effect
	chloral hydrate	Increases anticoagulant effect
	cholestyramine	Decreases warfarin absorption
	clofibrate	Increases anticoagulant effect
	corticosteroid	Increases anticoagulant effect
	dextrothyroxine	Increases anticoagulant effect
	glutethimide	Decreases anticoagulant effect
	mefenamic acid	Increases anticoagulant effect
	neomycin	Increases anticoagulant effect
	oxyphenbutazone	Increases anticoagulant effect
	phenylbutazone	Increases anticoagulant effect
	phenytoin	Increases phenytoin effects with bishydroxycoumarin; increases anticoagulant effect
	sulfonylurea	Increases sulfonylureas and anticoagulant effects
	thyroid preparation	Increases anticoagulant effect
	Vitamin K food or supplement	Decreases anticoagulant effect

because they increase the risk of hemorrhage. That risk must be weighed against the possible consequences of thrombosis or embolization. The possible contraindications:

1. moderate to severe hypertension (because of the increased likelihood of central nervous system hemorrhage)
2. hepatic or renal disease
3. last trimester of pregnancy (contraindicated for any anti-coagulant except heparin, which does not cross the placental barrier)
4. immediate postpartum period
5. severe diabetes
6. infections
7. pericarditis
8. severe head, bone, or muscle trauma associated with large, raw surfaces
9. aspirin intake.

Making sure a patient's within therapeutic range takes careful monitoring. Inadequate lab facilities or poor patient cooperation, therefore, are contraindications to anticoagulant therapy. So are senility and emotional instability, including chronic alcoholism, unless the dosage can be controlled by another person such as a family member.

Managing toxicities and side effects

Short-term heparin therapy rarely causes side effects except possible hemorrhage that can be major, or as minor as local ecchymoses. The risk is higher in women over 60. Bleeding from superficial wounds is less likely with heparin than with coumarin derivatives, but you must still remain alert for evidence of hemorrhage. If chills or spontaneous bleeding occur, withdraw the drug immediately.

Patients taking heparin rarely develop hypersensitivity reactions. But when a patient has a history of other drug allergies, the doctor may give him a trial dose of 1000 units to gauge his reaction before beginning standard therapy. A few patients do develop allergic reactions such as hyperemia, itching of the skin and mucous membranes, urticaria, asthma symptoms and, very rarely, anaphylaxis. Some patients report transient hair loss several months after therapy. A few suffer osteoporosis and spontaneous fractures after high doses of heparin taken for 6 months or longer.

You can usually manage a heparin overdose by simply

TIME SPAN OF DRUG ACTION

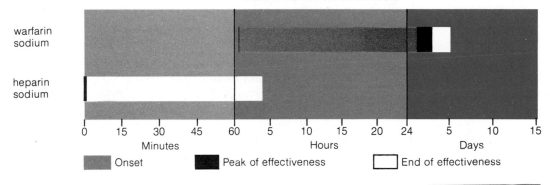

stopping therapy. In critical situations, use protamine sulfate to antagonize the effects of heparin quickly. Protamine sulfate works because, as a strong base, it reacts strongly with the acidic heparin to neutralize its action. Administer protamine sulfate with a slow I.V. and adjust the dose carefully, since it's a mild anticoagulant itself. A rule of thumb for dosage: 1 mg protamine sulfate will counteract the anticoagulant effect of approximately 100 units of heparin. If you have just given the heparin, use a full 1 mg of protamine sulfate per 100 units of heparin. If an hour has elapsed since the heparin injection, you'll need only ½ mg protamine sulfate per 100 units heparin because of the anticoagulant's 60-minute half-life.

As with heparin, the most serious side effect of oral anticoagulants is hemorrhage. It develops even with prescribed maintenance doses, so frequent blood tests are essential. It can develop in mucous membranes, skin, or gastrointestinal or genitourinary tracts. Hemorrhage is usually mild — but it can be severe, even fatal, from an unsuspected peptic ulcer. Watch for bruises, nosebleeds, and bleeding gums, all early signs of a bleeding tendency.

Coumarin derivatives can occasionally cause gastrointestinal reactions such as diarrhea and allergic reactions. They can be managed easily.

Some reports say blood clot formation will increase if you withdraw oral anticoagulants abruptly after long-term use; others disagree. Even so, a gradual reduction in dosage over several weeks may be wise.

For a coumarin overdose, doctors give vitamin K_1, about 5-10 mg orally, or 10-15 mg at 5 mg per minute I.V. However,

Dosage tip
A hospital patient on heparin is usually switched to an oral anticoagulant before he is discharged. Since oral anticoagulants take time to have their effect, remember to explain to the patient that he'll continue on heparin as well, for up to five days.

I.V. administration of vitamin K₁ is riskier because it may induce hypotension; oral vitamin K₁ is usually sufficient to manage overdosage.

The intramuscular route isn't good for coumarin overdosage. Oral vitamin K₁ controls mild bleeding, whereas I.V. K₁ is probably better for moderate to severe bleeding. After the patient receives vitamin K₁, he may be refractory to anticoagulants for several days or even weeks.

Blood or plasma transfusions will also antagonize the oral anticoagulants. This treatment may be needed when bleeding persists or blood replacement is necessary.

The trouble in adjusting the dosage of anticoagulants can stem partly from drug interactions. Remember, your cardiac patient may be given more than a dozen different drugs during hospitalization. Stress the dangers of interactions when teaching your patient about anticoagulant therapy. (For a list of these interactions, see the chart on page 111).

The key to success
To help your patient follow anticoagulant therapy, you'll teach the do's and don'ts, making sure to relate his therapy to his particular problem. When he shows that he's ready to learn, explain how blood clots can endanger his life and how anticoagulants will protect him from the dangers he may face.

To understand what you can do, consider the following case: Jane Venthom was about to be discharged from the hospital after surgery for the replacement of a mitral valve. Her nurse explained that she'd be on anticoagulant therapy for the rest of her life — to keep clots from forming on her new valve. Jane understood that she'd need frequent blood tests to make sure that her warfarin dosage was within therapeutic range. Her nurse showed her how to schedule her pills, so that she'd have no trouble remembering her medication. For a while, everything worked out well. But then Jane's prothrombin times became dangerously prolonged, subjecting her to the risk of massive hemorrhage. Talking to Jane, the nurse found out that she had been taking more than 2 grams of aspirin — and not considering such a common drug as "medicine," she'd not reported it. The nurse explained that aspirin increased the effect of her warfarin and that starting or stopping any medication without consulting her doctor might actually threaten her life. Once Jane understood the delicacy of her therapy, her

PATIENT TEACHING AID			MONTH			
SUN	MON	TUE	WED	THUR	FRI	SAT
DOSAGE _____ mg	DOSAGE _____ mg	DOSAGE _____ mg	DOSAGE _____ mg	DOSAGE _____ mg	DOSAGE _____ mg	DOSAGE _____ mg
DOSAGE _____ mg	DOSAGE _____ mg	DOSAGE _____ mg	DOSAGE _____ mg	DOSAGE _____ mg	DOSAGE _____ mg	DOSAGE _____ mg
DOSAGE _____ mg	DOSAGE _____ mg	DOSAGE _____ mg	DOSAGE _____ mg	DOSAGE _____ mg	DOSAGE _____ mg	DOSAGE _____ mg
DOSAGE _____ mg	DOSAGE _____ mg	DOSAGE _____ mg	DOSAGE _____ mg	DOSAGE _____ mg	DOSAGE _____ mg	DOSAGE _____ mg
DOSAGE _____ mg	DOSAGE _____ mg	DOSAGE _____ mg	DOSAGE _____ mg	DOSAGE _____ mg	DOSAGE _____ mg	DOSAGE _____ mg

prothrombin times returned to within therapeutic range, and she had no further problems.

You can help your patients avoid the risk Jane faced. Explain that all anticoagulant tablets aren't the same. "They vary in color, strength, and design," you should say. "Some are scored, others are not." Teach your patient to make up his dose by milligrams rather than by individual pills. Make sure he knows that periodically his dose may need to change if his clotting times and lab results change.

Explain drug interactions: This information is vital to your patient's safety. For the same reasons, he should understand the effects his diet will have on his therapy. Have him maintain his present diet but avoid foods high in vitamin K, such as yellow and green vegetables like broccoli, and high in fat, which increase the body's absorption of vitamin K. Since vomiting and diarrhea decrease absorption of oral anticoagulants, he should immediately report such conditions to his doctor. He may want to adjust his dosage temporarily. Alcohol has a variable effect on warfarin. Explain that drinking

Marking time
Patients taking anticoagulants can use calendars like the one above as a drug diary and a handy reminder to take their medicine. It shows the colors of all warfarin pills of various dosages and is available from Endo Laboratories, Inc., 1000 Steward Avenue, Garden City, New York 11530.

can increase the risks of gastritis, hemorrhage, and other complications.

Patients on anticoagulants should learn tips on safety. But be careful how you discuss these, since a frightened patient may stop therapy altogether. Suggest the following:

• Wear a Medic Alert bracelet and inform your dentist and other medical advisors that you're taking anticoagulants.

• Wear gloves while gardening. Use sharp items like knives cautiously. Don't use power tools or razors — try an electric shaver instead. And never trim corns, calluses or nails with a sharp knife or razor.

• Don't go barefoot.

• Don't take any other drugs, including over-the-counter preparations, without asking the doctor first. Don't make substitutions in drugs he has given you permission to take.

• Ask the doctor if you can drink alcohol.

• Don't use bath oils, which might cause you to slip in the tub. Place a nonslip bathmat in your tub for greater safety.

• Use a soft-bristle toothbrush rather than an electric toothbrush or a Water Pik.

• Don't play contact sports that might subject you to injury.

• Have a regular dental checkup to insure mouth hygiene and avoid disease.

Teach patients with thrombophlebitis how to dorsiflex their toes when at rest to increase the venous return from their legs. Show them how to wear elastic stockings, and then have them demonstrate. Stockings should be put on before rising from bed and taken off just before retiring at night. Make sure they avoid crossing or dangling their legs which impairs venous return to the heart.

Women of childbearing age who take anticoagulants will need special counseling. Unlike heparin, warfarin crosses the placental barrier, causing the fetus a risk of fatal hemorrhage in utero. Even after the baby is born, warfarin will appear in the milk of a nursing mother, once again jeopardizing her baby's blood clotting. For this reason, doctors place pregnant and nursing women on heparin, which does not cross the placental barrier or enter their milk. Tell women on anticoagulants that they can still have children but they should contact their doctors as soon as they become pregnant. They will then need close observation, frequent blood tests, and counseling.

Women on oral anticoagulants who are at risk for emboli should not use oral contraceptives or intrauterine devices. IUDs can cause them to bleed internally. Discuss other options such as diaphragms, condoms, contraceptive foam or gels, the rhythm method, tubal ligation, or vasectomy.

Of course, an emergency may occur, despite precautions. Instruct your patient about danger signs and what to do. He should call his doctor if he discovers any of the following signs:

- nosebleeds
- bloody gums
- red or brown urine
- red or black, tarry feces
- cuts that won't stop bleeding
- blood-tinged sputum
- bruises that don't heal but enlarge instead
- excessive menstrual flow
- headaches or pain in the abdomen
- dizziness, faintness, or unexplained weakness.

The manner in which you instruct your patient is crucial. He will most likely be apprehensive at first about his therapy. You can allay much of this apprehension by giving him a patient teaching card that will explain what he has to know about his drug. Copy the one on page 117, if it's appropriate, or make up your own. Then discuss the information on it with the patient and his family.

If he seems particularly apprehensive about possible bleeding from accidental injuries, reassure him that, in most cases, he'll be able to stop the bleeding by applying direct pressure to the cut. But, be sure to tell him that clotting may take a little longer than usual.

Discussing feelings

Always encourage the patient to discuss his feelings about his therapy. Watch for signs of depression, anxiety, or denial — all of which may affect his willingness to stay on his drug regimen. Try to include other family members in these discussions whenever possible, because they can offer reassurance and provide the patient with a support group.

You can help the patient get additional support by including him in group teaching sessions for patients on anticoagulant therapy. If your hospital doesn't have a program like this, ask your supervisor about starting one. Some hospitals have started programs successfully by scheduling classes for times when patients come for their blood tests.

Continued support and encouragement

Remember, your teaching role in anticoagulant therapy is vital to your patient's health. And what you've learned in this chapter will help you perform that role successfully. Provide reinforcement, encouragement, and support; three essentials for good patient education.

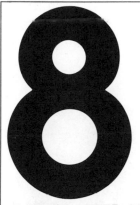

ANTILIPEMICS: Winning patient acceptance

BY FRANK F. WILLIAMS, PharmD

"MY FATHER WAS ONLY 40 years old when he died from a heart attack," Mr. DeLuca told the office nurse. Mr. DeLuca was a 37-year-old, overweight construction worker who'd come to the doctor for a checkup. His younger brother had died 2 months before from a heart attack, which prompted Mr. DeLuca to make an appointment. Autopsy reports revealed that both victims had atherosclerosis, and Mr. DeLuca was naturally afraid he'd get the same thing.

Seeing his doctor was prudent. When Mr. DeLuca's serum cholesterol and triglyceride levels were measured, he was found to have Type II hypercholesteremia. This condition increased his chances of developing atherosclerosis, as did his obesity and family history. The doctor couldn't change Mr. DeLuca's familial predisposition to the disease. But he could attempt to control the other two factors. He put Mr. DeLuca on a fat-controlled, reducing diet and gave him choles-tyramine, an antilipemic drug.

You'll hear how Mr. DeLuca fared on his therapy later on in this chapter. But first, let's look at atherosclerosis, considered by some to be the nation's number one health problem. Atherosclerotic plaques, which are accumulations of lipids

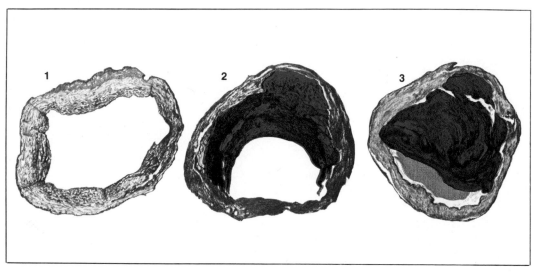

Lethal lipids
As atherosclerosis develops, a normal coronary artery (Figure 1) becomes roughened and narrowed by lipid deposits (Figure 2). If a blood clot develops, it may clog the artery (Figure 3), depriving the heart of its blood supply and causing a heart attack.

(fat-like material), are in everyone's blood vessels. They can eventually occlude the vessels and cause death from heart attack or stroke. In fact, cardiovascular disease from atherosclerosis is considered to be the leading cause of death in the United States.

What causes atherosclerosis? No one's sure. However, high risk factors have been identified: high blood lipid levels, cigarette smoking, hypertension, diabetes, overweight, lack of exercise, inherited predisposition, and possibly emotional stress. The more risk factors in a patient, the greater his chance of atherosclerosis — and maybe heart attack or stroke.

Current attempts to prevent or treat atherosclerosis are aimed at these risk factors. Mr. DeLuca, for example, was treated with antilipemic drugs and a fat-controlled diet to lower his lipid levels and reduce his weight.

By lowering cholesterol and triglyceride lipid levels to normal, the doctor hopes to lessen the patient's chance of cardiovascular disease by achieving the following:
 • Prevent the formation or enlargement of atherosclerotic plaques.
 • Decrease the size of existing plaques.

Whether this helps is uncertain, however. No proof exists that lowering lipid levels prevents heart disease. In fact, the FDA has put the following warning on all lipid-lowering drugs: "It has not been established whether the drug-induced lowering of serum cholesterol or triglyceride levels has a beneficial

TYPES OF HYPERLIPOPROTEINEMIA			
TYPE	NAME	FREQUENCY	POSSIBLE TREATMENTS
I	Fat-induced hyperlipemia	Rare	Very low-fat diet
II	Familial hyper-cholesteremia	Very common	Fat-controlled diet; cholestyramine
III	Hyperlipemia with abnormal beta-lipoproteins	Rare	Low-calorie diet if overweight; fat-controlled diet; clofibrate
IV	Carbohydrate-induced hyperlipemia	Very common	Low-calorie diet if overweight; fat-controlled diet; clofibrate
V	Mixed hyperlipemia	Uncommon	Diet low in cholesterol, fat, and carbohydrates; clofibrate or (experimental) estrogen

effect, no effect, or a detrimental effect on the morbidity or mortality due to atherosclerosis including coronary heart disease. Current investigations now in progress may yield an answer to this question."

However, let's suppose the doctor decides to treat a patient with antilipemic drugs and a fat-controlled, reducing diet. Your problem as a nurse will be twofold: teaching the patient about his drugs and helping him stay on his diet. This may be difficult at times — because you can't honestly say that failure to cooperate with therapy will *cause* heart disease, nor that compliance will *prevent* it. But you can encourage the patient to eliminate hyperlipidemia and obesity as risk factors — a worthwhile goal in his fight against heart disease.

Matching patient to therapy
Before the doctor can choose the right drug and diet to treat the patient, he must:

• Classify the hyperlipoproteinemia by type. This is usually done by measuring plasma cholesterol and triglyceride levels and inspecting the appearance of the serum after it's been refrigerated for 12 to 24 hours. Electrophoresis, or less frequently ultra-centrifugation, is needed for a more precise diagnosis.

• Rule out underlying disease as a cause. For example, diabetes, liver disease, nephrotic syndrome, certain dysglobulinemias, and the use of oral contraceptives.

	FOODS INCLUDED	FOODS EXCLUDED
BEVERAGES (NONDAIRY)	II—Coffee, tea, carbonated beverages, fruit and vegetable juices IV—Same as above, but only unsweetened beverages allowed	II—None IV—Sweetened beverages
BREADS AND CEREALS	II, IV—Enriched varieties of all breads except egg bread, saltines, and graham crackers. Baked goods containing no whole milk or egg yolks (angel food cake). All cereals and grain products (rice, macaroni, noodles, spaghetti) II—4 or more servings/day IV—Number of servings specified for weight control	II, IV—Biscuits, muffins, corn bread, pancakes, waffles, French toast, hot rolls, sweet rolls, corn or potato chips, flavored crackers
DAIRY PRODUCTS	II—Skim milk, nonfat buttermilk, evaporated skim milk, dried skim milk, uncreamed (no fat) cottage cheese, cheese made from skim milk plus specially prepared cheese high in polyunsaturated fat; ¼ cup creamed cottage cheese may be substituted for 1 oz meat IV—Same as above except that 2 oz of any cheese allowed per week	II, IV—Fresh, dried, evaporated or condensed whole milk; sweet or sour cream; yogurt; ice cream or ice milk; sherbet; commercial whipped toppings; cream cheese and all other cheese, except skim milk cheese; nondairy or other cream substitutes with exceptions shown under foods included
DESSERTS	II, IV—Angel food cake, puddings or frozen desserts made with skim milk, jello, meringues, fruit ices or whips, plus desserts made with allowed fats	II, IV—All cake and cookie mixes, except angel food mix; any pies, cakes, cookies containing whole milk, fat, or egg yolks; allowed fats included
FAT	II—Safflower oil, corn oil, soft safflower margarine, commercial mayonnaise IV—Any liquid vegetable unsaturated fat (safflower, corn, cottonseed, olive, and peanut oils), commercial mayonnaise, commercial salad dressings containing no sour cream or cheese	II—Butter, lard, hydrogenated shortening, and margarine; coconut oil and other oils not listed; salt pork, suet, bacon and meat drippings, gravies and sauces unless made with allowed fats and skim milk IV—Same as for II, except margarine made from unsaturated fat permitted
FRUITS	II—Any fresh, frozen, canned or dried fruit or juice of which 1 serving/day should be citrus fruit; avocado in small amounts 2 servings/day IV—Same as for II, except 3 servings/day and small amounts of avocado allowed	II, IV—None

PATIENT TEACHING AID
SPECIFIC DIETS FOR TYPE II, IV HYPERLIPOPROTEINEMIA

	FOODS INCLUDED	FOODS EXCLUDED
MEAT	II—Lean meat with fat trimmed off. Beef (ground round or chuck hamburger, roasts, pot roast, stew, steak, dried chipped beef), lamb, pork, ham, veal. Limit to 9 oz cooked/day including fish and poultry. Limit beef, lamb, ham, and pork to 3 oz portion 3 times/week IV—Same as for II except limit to 6-9 oz cooked/day	II—Fried meats, fatty meats such as bacon, cold cuts, hot dogs, luncheon meats, sausage, canned meats (e.g., Spam); corned beef, pork and beans, spareribs; commercially sold ground beef or hamburgers; meats canned or frozen in sauces or gravy; frozen or packaged prepared products. All organ meats, kidney, hearts, brains, liver, sweetbreads IV—Same as above minus all organ meats
POULTRY, FISH, AND EGGS	II—Skinned turkey, chicken or cornish hen; fish, water-packed tuna or salmon, limited amounts of shellfish (crab, clams, lobster, oysters, scallops) IV—Same as for II, except 3 egg yolks/week may be substituted for 2 oz shell fish or 2 oz organ meats; shrimp allowed	II—Poultry skin, fish canned in oil, goose, duck, fried poultry or fish, fish roe, including caviar IV—Same as above except for egg yolks and shrimp
SOUPS	II, IV—Bouillon, clear broth; any fat-free soups, cream soup made with skim milk, packaged broth-base dehydrated soups	II, IV—All others
SWEETS	II—Hard candies, jams, jelly, honey, sugar IV—Most concentrated sweets eliminated	II—Chocolate, all other candy IV—All candy, chocolate, jams, jelly, syrups, honey, sugar
VEGETABLES	II—2 to 4 servings/day of any vegetable (at least one dark green and one deep yellow vegetable daily) prepared with allowed fats IV—Same as for II, except limit amounts of potato, corn, lima beans, dried peas, and beans	II—Buttered, creamed, or fried vegetables except when prepared with safflower or corn oil IV—Same as for II, except when prepared with unsaturated fats
MISCELLANEOUS	II, IV—Pickles, salt, spice, herbs, vinegar, mustard, soy sauce, Worcestershire sauce plus nuts except those excluded, cocoa, peanut butter, olives	II, IV—Coconut, cashew and macadamia nuts, chocolate

As you can see on page 121, the most common types of hyperlipoproteinemia are Types II and IV. No matter which type the patient is, the doctor usually attempts to lower his lipid levels and reduce weight — if necessary — with the proper diet (see pages 122-123).

If this fails, he may prescribe an antilipemic drug, any of which lower cholesterol and/or triglycerides in most patients. How these drugs work varies from drug to drug, though most require a month to produce an effect. After that, the patient is checked once a month for 6 months to determine his progress, to adjust his dosage if necessary, and watch for undesirable side effects.

The antilipemics: clofibrate

Clofibrate is used to lower triglycerides and cholesterol in patients with Type III and IV hyperlipoproteinemia. Exactly how it works is not known, but it evidently inhibits cholesterol and triglyceride synthesis.

Warn the patients taking clofibrate that they may gain weight, become nauseated, or have abdominal discomfort. Men may have breast tenderness and a decreased libido. Uncommon side effects include dry skin, brittle hair, alopecia, skin eruptions, and muscle stiffness. Patients with kidney impairment may show an increased creatine phosphokinase.

If the patient is also taking an oral anticoagulant, he must be monitored closely and the dosage of his anticoagulant reduced by 50% to prevent bleeding (see drug interaction chart, page 127).

Niacin

Niacin lowers both cholesterol and triglyceride levels by inhibiting lipolysis in fat tissue and decreasing cholesterol synthesis.

Niacin's big disadvantage, however, is its many side effects. A patient may become flushed within 1 to 2 hours after taking it, but he can minimize this by eating something immediately after the dosage. Warn him of possible skin reactions: dry skin and increased pigmentation, especially in the groin and axilla. He may also have nausea, diarrhea, abdominal pain, increased urinary frequency, dysuria, and aggravation of peptic ulcer. Doses above 3 grams daily may impair liver function and cause jaundice. Niacin should be given cautiously to patients with

NURSES' GUIDE TO
ANTILIPEMICS

GENERIC NAME	TRADE NAME	ROUTE AND DOSAGE	COMMON SIDE EFFECTS
probucol	Loreico◇	P.O.: 500 mg 2 times a day	Diarrhea, flatulence, nausea, abdominal pain, vomiting hyperhydrosis
clofibrate	Atromid-S Liprinal◇◇	P.O.: 2 G daily in divided doses	GI disturbances, "flu-like" symptoms, cardiac arrhythmias, alopecia, urticaria, leukopenia, fatigue, headache, weight gain, decreased libido, increased SGOT, CPK, SGPT, proteinuria
sitosterols	Cytellin	P.O. (solution): 3 G before meals; up to 24-36 G a day	Bulky light-colored stools, mild laxative effect, flatulence, nausea, diarrhea
sodium dextrothyroxine	Choloxin	P.O.: initial dose 1-2 mg daily. Increase in 1-2 mg increments at monthly intervals to maintenance dose of 4-8 mg daily. Alter regimes for patients with abnormal thyroid functions	Angina pectoris, arrhythmias, ischemic myocardial changes, increase in heart size, insomnia, palpitations, tremors, weight loss, menstrual irregularities, GI disturbances, headache, tinnitus, dizziness, peripheral edema, visual disturbances, psychic changes, skin rashes
cholestyramine	Questran	P.O. (suspension): 4 G t.i.d. before meals. Maintenance dose 4 G t.i.d. before meals or q.i.d. before meals and before bed	Constipation (predisposing factors: dose greater than 24 G/day and age greater than 60 years), anorexia, bleeding tendencies, rash, osteoporosis
niacin	Niacin◇	P.O.: ½-3 G with or following meals	Generalized flushing, activation of peptic ulcers, jaundice, GI disturbances, dry skin and rash, dysuria, increased skin pigmentation, pruritus, hypotension, transient headache, tingling, decreased GTT, increased uric acid blood level
niacin (time released)	Nicobid	P.O.: 125-250 mg b.i.d. (a.m. and p.m.)	
colestipol hydrochloride	Colestid	P.O. (liquids): 15-30 G a day in 2-4 divided doses	Constipation, high levels of triglycerides

gout, because it increases uric acid levels; and to patients with diabetes, because it decreases glucose tolerance.

Cholestyramine

Cholestyramine decreases cholesterol levels by binding bile and acids in the gastrointestinal tract, preventing reabsorption. This increases bile acid production and turnover. Many doctors prefer it for patients with Type II hyperlipoproteinemia, because it lowers cholesterol by 20% to 25%.

However, cholestyramine has disadvantages: It can cause excessive gas production, and constipation. For the patient with these side effects, suggest a stool softener, like dioctyl sodium sulfosuccinate. The patient with an ileal bypass or malabsorption shouldn't take the drug. Cholestyramine's interactions with other drugs is shown on opposite page.

Another disadvantage to this drug is its taste. Because it must be mixed with liquid, many patients quit taking it. Prevent this from happening by suggesting liquids that disguise the drug's unpleasant taste: lemonade, orange juice, soda, or a semiliquid like applesauce.

Beta sitosterol

Beta sitosterol lowers cholesterol levels, probably by interfering with its absorption. It's a second-line drug for treating Type II hyperlipoproteinemia. Like cholestyramine, it can cause flatulence. It can also cause nausea and diarrhea.

To improve its taste, which is unpleasant, instruct the patient to mix it with chilled fruit juice.

Colestipol

Colestipol is also like cholestyramine in many ways: it lowers cholesterol levels by increasing bile acid production, and it produces the same side effects and drug interactions.

Like cholestyramine, it's unpleasant to take, because it must be mixed with liquids and doesn't dissolve. Help patients solve this by suggesting that they mix the drug with chilled applesauce, gelatin, or ice cream.

Sodium dextrothyroxine

Sodium dextrothyroxine benefits Type II and some Type IV patients by decreasing cholesterol and, to a lesser degree, triglyceride levels. However, it's contraindicated for patients

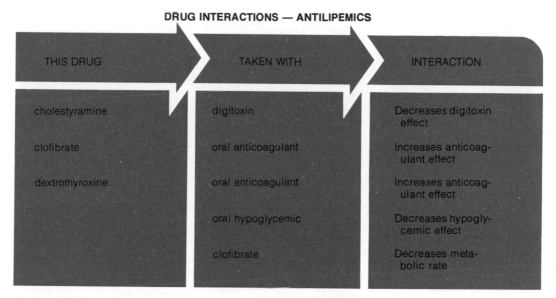

DRUG INTERACTIONS — ANTILIPEMICS

THIS DRUG	TAKEN WITH	INTERACTION
cholestyramine	digitoxin	Decreases digitoxin effect
clofibrate	oral anticoagulant	Increases anticoagulant effect
dextrothyroxine	oral anticoagulant	Increases anticoagulant effect
	oral hypoglycemic	Decreases hypoglycemic effect
	clofibrate	Decreases metabolic rate

who've had previous myocardial infarctions. In a recent study, those receiving this drug had a higher mortality rate than those receiving other antilipemic drugs. Other patients who can't take this drug are those with diabetes, hypertension, and advanced kidney or liver disease. Occasionally, a patient's metabolic rate will increase from this drug. For details on its interaction with other drugs, for example, anticoagulants — see the interaction chart above.

Probucol
Probucol lowers cholesterol levels by approximately 20%, but has little effect on triglyceride levels. It helps patients with Type II hyperlipoproteinemia, but — like most other antilipemics — causes many side effects. Some of the most common: diarrhea, flatulence, abdominal pain, nausea, and vomiting. Less frequently reported: excessive sweating, fetid sweat and angioneurotic edema.

Helping Mr. DeLuca
As you remember from earlier in this chapter, Mr. DeLuca's diagnosis was Type II hypercholesteremia. His doctor put him on a fat-controlled, reducing diet and 4 grams of cholestyramine twice a day.

How did he do? Well, like many patients, he balked at the

diet restrictions at first and objected to the taste of cholestyramine. The office nurse, however, was skilled at helping
patients on antilipemic drugs. She used the following
guidelines to encourage Mr. DeLuca to stay on his therapy —
and you can use them, too, in the hospital or office:

• Explain the need for therapy. Reinforce the importance of
controlling every possible risk factor.

• Discuss the drug's side effects and show ways to relieve
uncomfortable symptoms. Suggest alternate liquids with
which to mix the drug, if it tastes unpleasant.

• Supply the patient with sample menus and recipes to make
a fat-controlled diet more palatable. These are available at
bookstores, or you can write to Standard Brands, Inc., 625
Madison Avenue, New York, New York 10022 for the free
booklet "Sensible Eating Can Be Delicious." You can also
copy the helpful suggestions for food shopping and meal preparation that are in the appendices.

Spending time to review all these points with the patient
may tip the scales in his favor by keeping him on his drug
regimen and diet. With a patient like Mr. DeLuca, your efforts
could be the deciding factor. You could keep him from becoming another statistic in the yearly toll of heart disease victims.

SKILLCHECK 3

1. Maria Paone is an overweight 38-year-old housewife with moderate hypertension. For over a year, the doctor has controlled it effectively with reserpine. When you check Mrs. Paone's blood pressure today, it is 150/98. However, when she steps on the scale to be weighed, she confides that she'll soon be gaining even more weight. You ask why, and Mrs. Paone says she thinks she is pregnant. If she is, what effect could this have on her condition?

2. Rosie Salvatore, a plump 56-year-old, is an excellent cook. She is proud that her family delights in her Sunday dinners, and she tells you that her favorite activities are food shopping, cooking, and baking. Is it any wonder that she becomes upset when the doctor puts her on a fat-controlled diet to reduce her weight and serum lipid levels? Through her tears, Mrs. Salvatore tells you that she cannot exist on such a diet. How can you help her?

3. You've been working in a doctor's office for about a year. During that time, Mrs. Lottie Gottwald, a 46-year-old saleslady, has been in many times for blood pressure checks. She has essential hypertension, which the doctor has controlled with oral hydralazine. However, now Mrs. Gottwald tells you she thinks she has arthritis. In fact, her joints ache so much she may have to quit her job. What do you think the doctor will do?

4. Peter VanZandt, a 42-year-old securities analyst, is admitted to the CCU with a tentative diagnosis of acute myocardial infarction. This is confirmed by EKG and enzyme studies, and the doctor orders heparin 5000 units I.V. every six hours. He's still on anticoagulant therapy when he's transferred to your unit. When you measure his urine, you notice that it's slightly cloudy. What do you do?

5. Frank Rooney's serum lipid levels are high. He's a 60-year-old pipefitter with a family history of stroke. To reduce his risk of having one, Mr. Rooney takes cholestyramine, is on a fat-controlled diet, and has his blood checked regularly for serum lipid levels. When he comes in for his monthly checkup and you ask him how he is, he complains of constipation and gas. Do you know why?

6. James LaBarr, a 61-year-old used car salesman, is taking guanethidine to control his malignant hypertension. Two days ago, his doctor increased his dosage. This morning, Mr. LaBarr's wife rushed him to the emergency ward because he almost fainted when he got out of bed. You check his blood pressure, after he lies down on the examination table, and it is 130/78. Do you know why Mr. LaBarr had a dizzy episode earlier?

7. Forty-five-year-old Sara Henrich, a hotel housekeeper, is admitted to your unit after having an acute coronary occlusion. She's given heparin for 4 days, then switched to an oral anticoagulant, warfarin. When you see the order in the medication kardex, it reads warfarin 2.5 mg P.O. It's a standard dose, but still you feel uneasy about it. Why? What do you do?

8. Peter Lawler, a 55-year-old auto mechanic, has been taking warfarin for one week. He was admitted to the hospital with pulmonary embolism and is on complete bed rest. One morning when you are shaving him, you accidentally nick his chin. The cut bleeds profusely and Mr. Lawler naturally becomes quite upset. What do you do to stop the bleeding and how can you reassure Mr. Lawler?

9. Mabel Hegsted, a 68-year-old delicatessen owner, has been slightly hypertensive for over 20 years. After trying out several other drugs to control her hypertension, the doctor orders clonidine and asks you to reinforce what he has told her about its use and side effects. What will you tell Mrs. Hegsted?

(Answers on page 167)

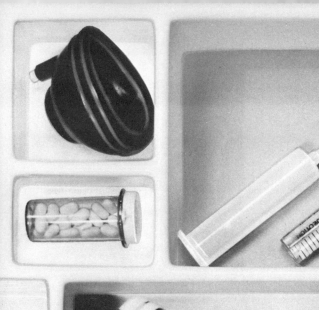
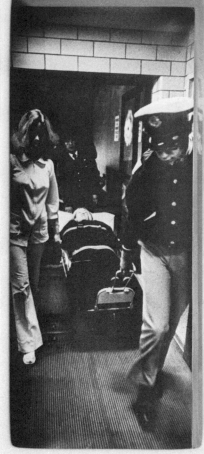
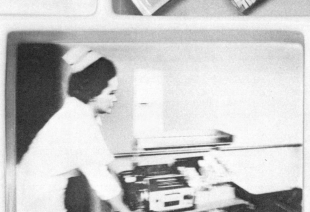
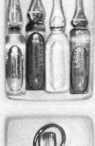

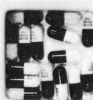
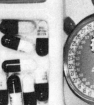
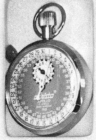
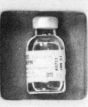
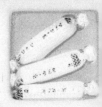
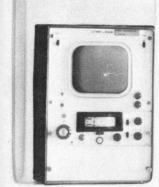
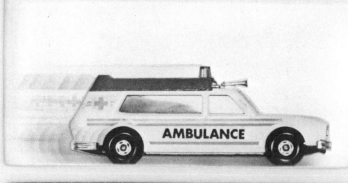

AMBULANCE

5% Dextrose

P363X̅... FEB 19
50 ml
5% Dextrose
Injection USP (5% Dextrose in Wa.er)

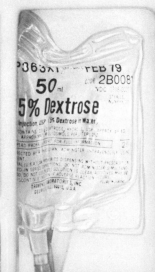
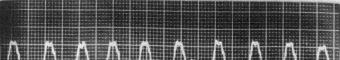

IN CASE OF EMERGENCY

Introducing the life-support drugs...
for use during a Code
or in hypertensive crisis.

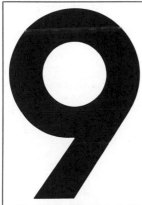

CPR DRUGS:
Supporting life
with definitive therapy

BY CATHERINE CIAVERELLI MANZI, RN

CODE 99...CODE BLUE...Code One...Code CRT. What do they mean? Cardiac emergency! One can happen anytime, anyplace — on a quiet morning in the doctor's office, late at night on the medical-surgical floor, during a routine test in a clinic lab.

Are you prepared for a cardiac emergency? A person's life may depend on your knowledge of basic cardiopulmonary resuscitation (CPR) and complicated CPR drug therapy. This chapter will hone your skills in this area and make you more valuable during the next code. You'll learn how CPR drugs work, how to save time organizing equipment and procedures, and how to save lives.

Take the case of 59-year-old Mrs. Jansen. She was waiting in her doctor's office for a routine physical one morning, when the nurse heard her cry out, saw her clutch her throat and collapse on the floor, unconscious. The nurse rushed to her side, found that Mrs. Jansen was not breathing, and had no carotid pulse. Without leaving her side, the nurse called for help and immediately began giving CPR — artificial respiration accompanied by external cardiac compression. When the doctor arrived, he administered the appropriate drugs to com-

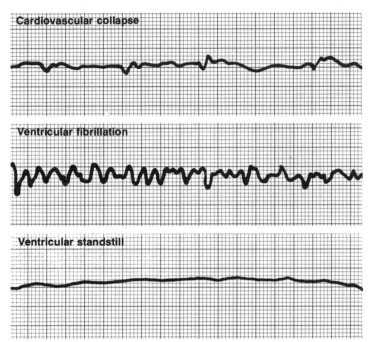

Cardiovascular collapse

Ventricular fibrillation

Ventricular standstill

plement the nurse's physical rescue efforts: They were sodium bicarbonate I.V. bolus to correct metabolic acidosis, and epinephrine to strengthen the myocardium. An EKG was hooked up to determine the type of cardiac arrest.

What kind of arrest?

Of course, not every case is like Mrs. Jansen's (you'll hear more about her later). That's because there's more than one kind of cardiac arrest, which — as you know — occurs when cardiac output is insufficient to sustain life. Here are three basic types:

• *Cardiovascular collapse*. An EKG will show the heart is still beating, but not strong enough to circulate an adequate amount of blood to the brain and other body tissues. Peripheral pulse is usually absent. This condition results from myocardial infarction or myocardial shock caused by severe hemorrhage, electrocution, drug or anesthetic overdosage, or drowning.

• *Ventricular fibrillation*. The heart beats wildly and ineffectively. Without synchronized contractions, cardiac output is nil, and there's no peripheral pulse or blood pressure. If you were to inspect the heart directly, it would look and feel like a bag of worms. This condition may occur after a myocardial infarction or low-voltage electrical shock.

• *Ventricular standstill (asystole)*. The heart has stopped beating. No mechanical or electrical activity shows on the EKG and pulse and blood pressure are absent. This condition is likely to be irreversible and usually means a severely anoxic myocardium.

Know life-support

All three types of cardiac arrest are emergencies and require immediate life-support measures. You can remember the order in which these measures are taken (in most cases) by remembering ABCD: A — airway opened; B — breathing restored (artificial respiration); C — circulation restored (external cardiac compression); D — definitive treatment (diagnosis, drugs, and defibrillation).

On page 136, Figures 1-4 illustrate some of the steps you must know for life support: the proper head tilt needed for an open airway, and the relationship of hands to heart during external cardiac compression. Figure 5 shows how you should position yourself to give effective CPR, which many times is done incorrectly by untrained personnel. You should learn CPR from a qualified teacher. If your hospital doesn't provide it, enroll in a course sponsored by the American Heart Association or American Red Cross.

By knowing the ABCs of life support, you're less likely to become confused or panicky. You'll be ready to help the doctor with the D step for life support: definitive treatment (diagnosis, drugs, and defibrillation). In most arrest cases, the doctor will supervise definitive treatment. But where pre-written drug and defibrillation protocols exist — as they do in many specialized units — you may be responsible.

Without extensive training, though, you won't be supervising emergency protocols on your own. However, we can help you understand why certain drugs are given and how to save precious seconds for the doctor giving them.

Sodium bicarbonate

Sodium bicarbonate is used to correct metabolic acidosis. This condition occurs when the body's oxygen supply dwindles during cardiac arrest or abnormally drops — as it does during

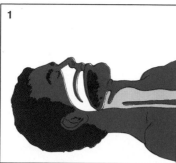

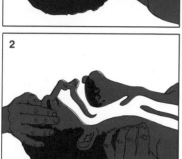

ABCs of CPR

To learn how to perform CPR properly, you must receive instruction from a qualified teacher. These pictures merely illustrate some of the steps involved in basic life support. For example, Figures 1 and 2 show how the head is tilted on an unconscious victim to relieve tongue obstruction and open the airway. Figures 3 and 4 show the proper relationship of hands to heart during external cardiac compression. Hands are placed two finger-widths above the tip of the xiphoid process to avoid lacerating liver. The lower half of the sternum is compressed 1½-2 inches with each downstroke. Figure 5 shows you the correct position to administer CPR, with knees close to victim's chest and victim placed on a hard surface. As you can see, keeping your arms straight and at a 90° angle to the victim's chest is essential.

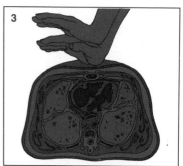

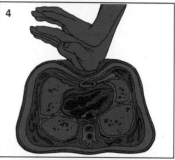

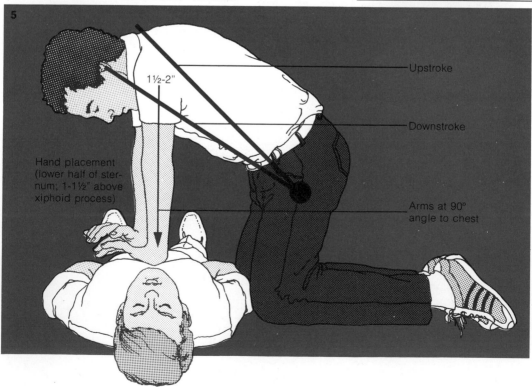

Upstroke

Downstroke

Hand placement (lower half of sternum; 1-1½" above xiphoid process)

1½-2"

Arms at 90° angle to chest

artificial respiration and artificial circulation. (Some acidosis may exist before the patient arrests; in fact, acidosis may be one of the causes of arrest.)

Metabolic acidosis depresses heart action and increases the risk of ventricular fibrillation. Because the myocardium doesn't respond well to drugs and defibrillation when acidotic, acidosis must be treated as quickly as possible. This is done by giving the patient frequent I.V. doses of sodium bicarbonate until effective respiration and circulation are restored or blood gas determinations dictate otherwise.

The initial sodium bicarbonate dose (as recommended by the American Heart Association) is 1 mEq/kg body weight. For example, a patient weighing 70 kg (154 pounds) would get 70 ml of an 8.4% solution which contains 1 mEq/ml. If the patient doesn't respond, the same dose should be repeated in 10 minutes. Further dosages should be based on arterial blood gas determinations. When these are not available, half the initial dose can be given at 10-minute intervals (see dosage chart page 138).

Blood gas and blood pH determinations are needed because too much sodium bicarbonate can cause alkalosis. This aggravates tissue hypoxia by causing a firmer bond of oxygen to hemoglobin making less oxygen available to vital tissues. Alkalosis and hypoxia — as well as acidosis — interfere with the restoration of normal sinus rhythm.

The fastest and most accurate way to give sodium bicarbonate is by bolus injection using prefilled, labeled, disposable syringes. However, sometimes it's given by I.V. infusion, using a 500 ml bottle of 5% solution, but this method has drawbacks. Other drugs, such as calcium chloride, are precipitated by sodium bicarbonate. Opening the sodium bicarbonate bottle before it's used causes a decrease in the bicarbonate concentration. The bottle also takes up valuable space on the I.V. pole.

What are sympathomimetics?
Sympathomimetics (epinephrine, dopamine, norepinephrine, isoproterenol, and metaraminol) are probably the most widely used drugs for resuscitation. As adrenergic drugs, they stimulate either alpha or beta receptors of the sympathetic nervous system. Some stimulate both receptors.

Alpha adrenergic stimulators cause arterial and venous con-

CPR for kids
CPR for infants and small children varies from that for adults as follows: (1) To compress the chest in children, use the heel of only one hand; in infants, use only the tips of two fingers. (2) Compress the midsternum in infants only ½-¾ inch; and in small children only ¾-1½ inch. (3) The rate of compressions to ventilations is 5:1, with 80-100 compressions a minute. Remember that infants and small children need only small breaths to inflate their lungs. (4) When you tilt a child's head back to open the airway, you also lift his back, so be sure you support his back carefully with your hand.

Remember, to learn how to perform CPR properly you must receive instruction from a qualified teacher.

NURSES' GUIDE TO
ESSENTIAL EMERGENCY DRUGS FOR RESUSCITATION

DRUG	ROUTE AND DOSAGE	EFFECTS AND USES
atropine sulfate	I.V. bolus, 0.5 mg, may repeat	Decreases vagal tone in pronounced bradycardia
calcium chloride	I.V. bolus, intracardiac 1 G (10 ml of a 10% solution), may repeat	Positive inotrope for asystole; increases force of contractions in a feebly beating heart
dopamine HCl (Intropin)	I.V. infusion at 5 mcg/Kg/min up to 20-50 mcg/Kg/min	Increases blood pressure and perfusion; maintains renal perfusion; positive inotropic effect; increases cardiac output
epinephrine HCl (Adrenalin)	I.V. bolus, intracardiac 0.5 to 1 mg (5 to 10 ml of a 1:10,000 solution), may repeat	Asystole, ventricular fibrillation (with bicarbonate); increases amplitude of fibrillatory waves, positive inotrope, positive chronotrope, peripheral vasoconstriction
isoproterenol (Isuprel)	I.V. bolus, intracardiac 0.2 mg I.V. infusion titrated to heart rate, blood pressure 2 mg/500 ml D₅W	Asystole, cardiovascular collapse; positive inotrope, positive chronotrope, increases cardiac output and blood pressure
lidocaine (Xylocaine)	I.V. bolus: 100 mg followed by I.V. infusion 1 to 2 G in 500 ml D₅W at 2 to 3 mg/min	Ventricular irritability, ventricular tachycardia, PVCs; raises fibrillation threshold
metaraminol (Aramine)	I.M.: 2-10 mg; I.V.: 15-100 mg in 500 D₅W/NSS	Vasopressor increases peripheral resistance, improves cardiac contractility and cardiac, cerebral, and renal blood flow.
norepinephrine levarterenol (Levophed)	I.V. infusion titrated to blood pressure, 2 to 4 ampuls in 500 ml D₅W	Vasopressor, increases peripheral pressure and perfusion.
sodium bicarbonate 50 mEq (8.4%, 50-ml solution)	I.V. bolus, 1 mEq/Kg initially, repeat in 10 minutes if necessary. Further doses based on blood gas analysis. If tests unavailable, use ½ initial dose every 10 minutes.	Reverse metabolic acidosis; facilitates defibrillation (with epinephrine)

striction, elevate blood pressure by increasing peripheral vascular resistance, decrease heart rate, and increase venous pooling.

Beta adrenergic stimulators cause skeletal muscle vessel dilation, elevate blood pressure, increase the heart rate by stimulating the SA node, strengthen contractions, and decrease venous pooling. For a full explanation of how drugs affect alpha and beta receptors, refer back to Chapter 1 for a review of the autonomic nervous system.

Before sympathomimetics can be effective, the following conditions need attention: plasma and blood volume deficits, electrolyte and pH abnormalities, and arrhythmias. Which drug is chosen depends partly on the patient's blood pressure. If it must be elevated immediately to get oxygen to the heart and brain, then a drug with potent vasoconstrictive properties is needed. Therapy would probably begin with norepinephrine or metaraminol, after acidosis has been corrected.

Epinephrine

This drug acts on both beta and alpha receptors, but primarily beta. It makes the heart beat faster and contract more forcefully, thus increasing cardiac output. It decreases peripheral vascular resistance by vasodilation, but it also has some vasoconstrictive properties. Epinephrine's action usually converts ventricular fibrillation from fine to coarse, and makes the heart more responsive to DC shock. Used with sodium bicarbonate and CPR, it can change a ventricular standstill to a rhythmic beat; or change a standstill to a fibrillation responsive to DC shock.

When epinephrine is given with sodium bicarbonate, it increases blood pressure and blood flow to the brain. However, it's inactivated by direct contact with sodium bicarbonate, so the two drugs should never come in contact with each other.

Dopamine

Another sympathomimetic drug that affects both alpha and beta receptors is dopamine. It acts as a vasoconstrictor on the skeletal muscle blood vessels, but dilates renal and mesenteric vessels. This has a positive inotropic effect on the myocardium, causing an increase in cardiac output, renal blood flow, glomerular infiltration, and urine production. However, these effects are dose related; high doses cause the opposite effects.

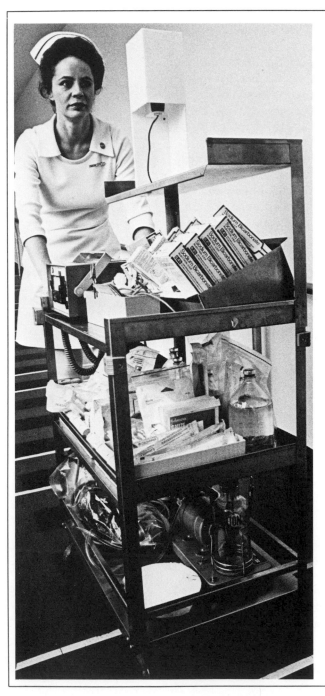

CONTENTS OF CPR CART

TOP SHELF: work space

SECOND SHELF:
defibrillator
Prepackaged drugs:
   sodium bicarbonate
   calcium chloride, 1 G
   epinephrine, 1 mg
   atropine, 1 mg
   isoproterenol, 2 mg ampul (infusion)
   isoproterenol, 0.2 mg bolus with
   10 ml syringe and 10 ml of diluent
   lidocaine, 100 mg bolus
   lidocaine, 1 G (for infusion)
   propranolol, 1 mg ampul
   hydrocortisone sod. succinate, 1 G
   levarterenol bitartrate, 4 cc
   dopamine, 200 mg ampul
I.V. solution: D_5W 500 cc
armboards (1 large, 1 medium)
EKG gel for defibrillation
EKG leads
alcohol sponges, tourniquets, I.V.
   additive labels, and alligator
   clip for pericardiocentesis

THIRD SHELF:
50 cc plastic syringes
10 cc plastic syringes (Luer tip)
3 and 5 cc plastic syringes with
   needles
EKG tape
intracaths — large only
16 and 18 gauge Jelco needles
16 and 18 gauge Medicuts
18, 20, and 21 gauge disposable
   needles
18 or 19 gauge 3" spinal needles
   (for I.C. use)
18 or 19 gauge 6" spinal needles
adhesive tape (½-1")
13 or 15 gauge 1½" disposable
   needle (for floating pacemaker)
2 blood sampling kits
minidropper sets
standard I.V. sets
suction catheters
O_2 connecting tubes
Levin stomach tube
airways (large and medium)
cut-down kit
3-0 silk with cutting needle
4" x 4" gauze pads

BOTTOM SHELF: aspirator, Ambu bag

Although dopamine is not usually a first-line CPR drug, you may find it on emergency carts for use in patients with shock. It works best in patients whose urine flow, myocardial function, and blood pressure have not deteriorated greatly.

It should not be given to patients with pheochromocytomas, uncorrected tachyarrhythmias, or ventricular fibrillation. Don't mix it with alkaline solutions; use D_5W, a saline solution, or a combination of D_5W and a saline solution.

By infiltrating surrounding tissue, dopamine can cause sloughing and necrosis near the injection site. To prevent this, start the I.V. in a large vein — preferably one in the antecubital fossa — not a vein in the hand, wrist, or ankle. Watch the site carefully. If drug infiltration occurs, stop the infusion immediately and call the doctor. He way want to counteract the dopamine's adverse effect with an injection of 10-15 ml normal saline and 5-10 mg of phentolamine. Should dopamine be discontinued, watch the patient closely for possible drop in blood pressure.

Depending on his response to dopamine, a patient may need his dosage adjusted. If his blood pressure elevates excessively, the dosage may have to be reduced or discontinued.

Norepinephrine
This drug acts primarily on alpha receptors. It decreases heart rate and cardiac output, despite the fact that it increases myocardial contractility. Norepinephrine also acts as a vasoconstrictor, increasing peripheral vascular resistance which increases systemic blood pressure.

Important drug interaction: If the patient has been taking reserpine, phenothiazines, or antidepressants prior to arrest, these drugs will inhibit norepinephrine's action.

Isoproterenol
This drug is a pure beta receptor stimulator, and has almost no effect on alpha receptors. It makes the heart beat faster and more forcefully, produces mild peripheral vasodilation, and increases cardiac output. It also relaxes the smooth muscle of the bronchioles.

Because isoproterenol can cause tachycardia, it must be used cautiously, and not at all if the patient has tachycardia from digitalis intoxication. Also, it must *not* be given simultaneously with epinephrine because both drugs are direct cardiac stimulants and together may produce serious arrhythmias. However, they may be given alternately.

Metaraminol

This drug acts primarily by releasing naturally occurring catecholamines from post-ganglionic nerve endings. It acts on alpha receptors in the arteries and beta receptors in the heart. In lower dosages, the drug's inotropic effect predominates, and this increases cardiac output. In higher doses, its effects are similar to those of norepinephrine.

Important drug interaction: If the patient has been taking reserpine or guanethidine prior to arrest, these drugs will inhibit metaraminol's action. The reason: They work by depleting catecholamines, leaving none for the metaraminol to release.

Calcium chloride or calcium gluconate

Though not classed as sympathomimetics, both of these drugs improve myocardial tone during CPR and make the heart contract more forcefully after a rhythmic EKG is restored. They also increase blood and pulse pressures and improve blood flow to the brain.

Lidocaine

This drug controls ventricular arrhythmias by depressing automaticity in the His-Purkinje network. It raises the electrical excitability threshold of the ventricle, thereby preventing discharge of an ectopic rhythm or premature beat. It has little or no effect on the atria, so it's not particularly useful for treating atrial arrhythmias and does not change myocardial contractility or blood pressure. (However, large doses of 5 mg or more per minute can decrease myocardial conduction.) Lidocaine penetrates cardiac tissue very rapidly and acts within 60 seconds after an I.V. bolus dose. Since the effect of a bolus dose only lasts 15 minutes, a continuous I.V. infusion must be started at the same time to maintain a therapeutic level of the drug. You can see how this works on the opposite page.

Lidocaine should not be used when there's a complete heart block. The reason: It may suppress or abolish the substitute pacemaker action in the ventricles that's maintaining the heart beat. This also applies when the sinoatrial node is depressed, as in sinoatrial block, sinus bradycardia, atrioventricular or

MAINTAINING THERAPEUTIC BLOOD LEVELS WITH LIDOCAINE

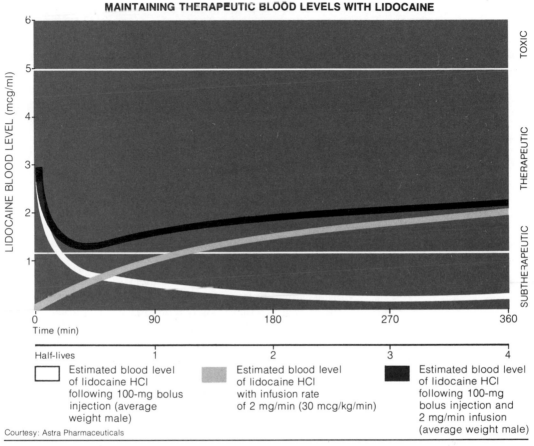

Courtesy: Astra Pharmaceuticals

Estimated blood level of lidocaine HCl following 100-mg bolus injection (average weight male)	Estimated blood level of lidocaine HCl with infusion rate of 2 mg/min (30 mcg/kg/min)	Estimated blood level of lidocaine HCl following 100-mg bolus injection and 2 mg/min infusion (average weight male)

intraventricular block.

Give lidocaine cautiously to patients with Adams-Stokes syndome, liver disease or congestive heart failure, because it may cause toxicity. Also, patients who are hypersensitive to local anesthetics should not get it.

Lidocaine can cause many side effects: convulsions, drowsiness, paresthesia, hearing difficulties, muscle twitching, slurred speech, agitation, confusion, nausea, and vomiting.

Always check each dose as you give it, and check the total dosage over a period of 8 hours. If the patient shows side effects, such as vomiting, or diarrhea, you may control these by reducing the infusion rate. If CNS side effects occur (agitation, confusion, paresthesia, slurred speech, drowsiness), *stop the infusion immediately* and call the doctor.

Lidocaine blood levels
This chart shows why both bolus injections and continuous I.V. infusion of lidocaine are needed to maintain therapeutic blood levels.

Atropine sulfate

Atropine increases heart rate by blocking parasympathetic activity on the SA node and AV junctional area. In patients with bradycardia and hypotension, it can increase blood pressure and cardiac output.

Always watch patients on atropine closely to determine the drug's effect on the heart rate. If it stays the same or decreases, the dosage may be too small (less than 0.3 mg), or the injection may have been given too slowly.

Never give atropine to patients with glaucoma, because it can cause an increase in intraocular pressure. It can also cause urinary retention, so it should be used with caution for patients with bladder problems. Other side effects include: mouth dryness and blurred vision. These last two effects are usually temporary.

What's your role in CPR?

You may lack the training to supervise definitive therapy during a code, but here are some important guidelines to help you, no matter what your responsibility:

• Know the ABCs of basic life support and how to give them.

• Make sure your unit, clinic, or office has a cart with the essential CPR drugs and equipment, as illustrated on page 140. See that someone is assigned to check the cart daily and after each code to (1) restock supplies and (2) check equipment to make sure it works and has all the necessary parts. *Drugs must not be allowed to expire.*

• If you're giving drugs during a code, use a large gauge I.V. catheter; a smaller one, such as a butterfly needle or a ½-1 inch catheter, could slip out of the vein wall and cause subcutaneous infiltration of the drug. Or it could penetrate the opposite wall of the vein and make it collapse. These risks are greatest when drugs are given at frequent intervals, or in large amounts. (If no I.V. is in place when an arrest occurs, start one as soon as you can, using D5W; you may have difficulty finding a vein later. In case the doctor decides to use a subclavian vein, have a CVP tray set up.)

• Keep track of which drugs are given, their dosages, and the time interval between dosages. Know why each drug is given, so you can tell if it's effective. Be aware of possible drug interactions and side effects.

• Know what drugs the doctor needs and have them opened

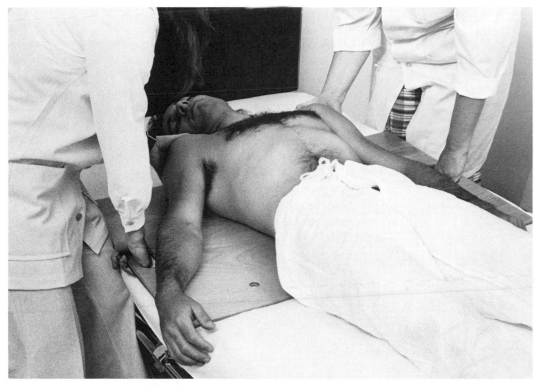

and ready when he asks for them. Have the defibrillator turned on and the paddles clean. Make sure gel is handy to coat paddles when needed. Do *not* coat them in advance.

• Be alert for changes in the patient's condition and know what's going on at all times. This includes checking to see if CPR is being given correctly, watching I.V. infusion rates, checking the patency of I.V. tubes, and observing the EKG monitor. Check the patient's carotid or femoral pulse. A strong pulse indicates adequate blood perfusion to vital organs and tissues. Look at the pupils — do they react to light? Note their size; if they are fixed and dilated and do not react to light, brain damage may have occurred.

• Don't panic. You'll function with greater efficiency if your mind is clear and focused on the immediate problem. Work as quickly as you can without undue haste.

Speed, accuracy, knowledge, and observation are crucial during any code. They were when Mrs. Jansen arrested that morning in her doctor's office. Fortunately, the nurse's CPR

Board stiff
What if you have an unconscious bedridden patient in need of CPR and you can't move him to a hard surface? Place a board, the full width of his bed if possible, under his chest so his body has the support it needs for effective cardiac compression. But don't delay giving CPR while waiting for the necessary support.

efforts and the doctor's drug therapy restored Mrs. Jansen's heart beat to a regular sinus rhythm (72 beats per minute) and her blood pressure to 130/76. She was transported by ambulance to the hospital where her arrest was diagnosed as a ventricular standstill (based on the EKG done in the office). She was placed in the CCU to determine the cause of her arrest, as well as to closely monitor her blood pressure, heart rate, and rhythm.

Will a patient under your care be as lucky as Mrs. Jansen if an arrest occurs? Perhaps...but probably not if you lack knowledge of basic life support measures. Be prepared: Review everything you've learned in this chapter and give the patient every chance to survive. What you take time to learn and remember today, may help you save a life tomorrow.

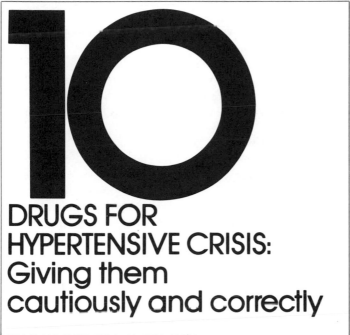

10
DRUGS FOR HYPERTENSIVE CRISIS:
Giving them cautiously and correctly

BY GAYLE WHITMAN, RN, BSN

EVERY NURSE KNOWS the danger of hypertensive crisis, and fortunately, we have drugs to remedy the crisis. But you must be careful of several things in giving those drugs: First, not to let the drugs overdo it — bring on hypotensive crisis…second, guard against their sometimes severe side effects…and third, follow the safest methods in administering them.

Consider the case of Simon Harris, a 42-year-old man with a history of long-standing hypertension. He was admitted to the E.R., accompanied by his wife. She said he'd been having headaches for the three days before and acting strangely — with decreased attention span, lack of concentration, and irritability. Mr. Harris' blood pressure measured 300/200.

He appeared confused and combative. Ophthalmic exam revealed retinal arteriolar spasms, exudates, and hemorrhages. Clinical diagnosis: acute hypertensive crisis with associated hypertensive encephalopathy.

We started an intra-arterial pressure line. Then we began nitroprusside, I.V., 25 mg/250 cc of D_5W and transferred Mr. Harris to the ICU. His pressure there remained elevated with a diastolic above 150 mm Hg. His neurologic status deteriorated: He developed rightsided hemiparesis and, then, a coma state. Drug therapy was switched to continuous infusion of trimethaphan 100 mg/liter.

Would you expect him to improve on this drug? Why? Were his admitting symptoms typical of hypertensive crisis? Before answering these questions, let's review the mechanisms of hypertensive crisis and the drugs commonly used to combat it.

Evaluating the patient
What precipitates a crisis like Mr. Harris'? We don't always know. Some patients with essential hypertension can develop a crisis if they become severely upset emotionally, or abruptly discontinue their antihypertensive drugs, or increase salt consumption...or simply don't get enough medication. Some patients with renal disease are prone to hypertensive crisis: those with acute or chronic glomerulonephritis, chronic pyelonephritis, or renal vascular disease. In them, perhaps the renin-angiotension mechanism somehow initiates the crisis.

Patients with pheochromocytoma (adrenal medullary tumor) are also prone to hypertensive crisis. This tumor manufactures and releases large amounts of epinephrine and norepinephrine. These periodically bombard the sympathetic nervous system, and elevate blood pressure.

Another group of patients prone to hypertensive crisis: those taking monamine oxidase (MAO) inhibitors such as tranylcypromine and isocarboxazid. These drugs, not used commonly nowadays, potentiate the action of sympatho-mimetic drugs such as levarterenol, dopamine, and others.

Hypertensive crisis begins with acute rise in diastolic blood pressure. Usually, diastolic readings over 120 mm Hg are dangerous; readings over 110 mm Hg are dangerous in pregnant women and children.

Pathologically, such levels of diastolic blood pressure produce acute vascular changes, mostly in the arterioles. The arterioles thicken and narrow. Necrotizing arteriolitis appears in the arterial wall, leading to damage of vital organs such as the kidney, heart, and brain. These necrotized arterioles may rupture and cause small hemorrhage into the organs. The aim of therapy: Lower blood pressure as rapidly as possible to prevent further damage.

The most severe complications of an accelerated hypertensive crisis — no matter what the cause of crisis — is hypertensive encephalopathy. It's almost inevitable at pressures

over 250/150 mm Hg. You'll observe its effects as severe
headaches, nausea, vomiting, mental confusion, convulsions,
visual disturbances, or nystagmus. Severe retinal arteriolar
spasm, visible through eyeground examination, probably re-
flect the state of arterioles in the brain. (See Chapter 6 for
eyeground photos).

Psychological changes include drowsiness, disorientation,
even stupor.

Even *moderate* hypertension can create an emergency if the
patient shows signs of acute left ventricular failure. Here, even
the stress of moderately increasing the left ventricle's work
proves too much.

Acute coronary insufficiency can also push up blood pressure. In this case, we don't know what's the precipitating
factor — the hypertension or the ischemia.

In two other conditions hypertension is considered an
emergency: (1) intracranial hemorrhage and (2) acute dissecting aneurysm. In the first, blood pressure must be lowered to
prevent further damage. In the second, blood pressure should
be maintained at a systolic level of 100-120 mm Hg to prevent
exsanguination.

Selecting the drug

Drugs for hypertensive crises generally fall into one of two
categories: vasodilators or sympathetic nervous system blocking agents.

The *vasodilators* include hydralazine, nitroprusside, and
diazoxide. All three decrease blood pressure by directly dilating vascular smooth muscles.

Drugs that block the sympathetic nervous system are:
trimethaphan camsylate (this blocks both sympathetic and
parasympathetic systems at the autonomic ganglia); reserpine; methyldopa; and phentolamine. (See Chapter 1 for an
explanation of how drugs work on the autonomic nervous
system.)

For a hypertensive crisis, these drugs are usually given I.V.
or I.M., because the oral route won't bring rapid enough
action.

• *Hydralazine* can be given either I.V. or I.M. If given I.V.,
the injection rate shouldn't exceed 0.5 ml/min. It should work
in 10 minutes. When it starts to lower the blood pressure,
adjust the injection frequently, lest hypotension develop.

TIME SPAN OF DRUG ACTION

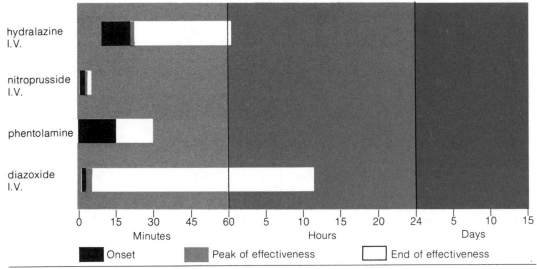

• *Nitroprusside* is given only I.V. Its action is instantaneous, and its effects last only 1-2 minutes after the drug is discontinued.

• *Phentolamine* works instantly, given I.V. It can also be given I.M. or as a single rapid I.V. bolus dose.

• *Diazoxide* acts more slowly than these two drugs — within 3-5 minutes after an I.V. bolus. The usual 300-600 mg bolus dose must be given as rapidly as possible (10-20 seconds at most) since the drug quickly binds with plasma protein, rendering it ineffective. Diazoxide's effects will usually last 4-12 hours.

• *Trimethaphan* also acts rapidly — usually within 2-5 minutes. It's given as I.V. infusion, with dosage regulated to blood pressure readings. Its effect lasts for 10-20 minutes after administration is discontinued.

• *Methyldopa* is given by I.V. infusion for hypertensive crisis over 30-60 minutes and can be repeated in 6 hours. Dose is titrated to blood pressure.

• *Reserpine* also acts slower, like methyldopa — within 2-3 hours. Its actions are less predictable, and that makes it a less likely choice for crisis. It's given I.M. or I.V.

Which drugs get used when? That depends on several things, including the reason for hypertensive crisis. Let's examine the major kinds of crisis, see what signs and symptoms

TIME SPAN OF DRUG ACTION

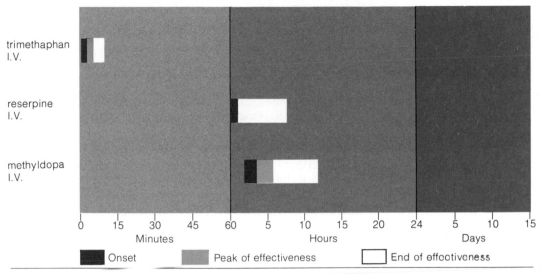

you should watch for, and learn what nursing interventions are needed for each crisis.

Acute hypertensive encephalopathy

Preferred drugs here are diazoxide, nitroprusside, and trimethaphan. Reserpine and methyldopa aren't used, because their side effect of drowsiness could mask neurologic signs. Moreover, they work too slowly for a crisis.

Trimethaphan can cause paralysis of pupillary reflex and accommodation of eye. So, routine pupil checks may be inaccurate if the patient's taking one of these drugs.

If you're giving nitroprusside, observe the following precautions. Before starting it, first ask the doctor what parameters he wants to achieve. Does he want a systolic below 90, or the drug titrated to hold the arterial mean at 80 mm Hg or below? Once this has been achieved, obtain baseline vital signs. If the patient has a CVP line, take a reading. If he has a low CVP reading, even small doses of nitroprusside could cause further vasodilation and a drop in blood pressure from hypovolemia.

Increase the dose of nitroprusside slowly and carefully; and at the same time, constantly monitor the blood pressure. If a CVP line isn't available, you must rely on clinical signs and symptoms. For example, are the patient's extremities warm, with good venous filling, or are they cold, indicating con-

Under wraps
Wrap nitroprusside in foil to prevent deterioration (see opposite page). Since the solution is unstable, a fresh one must be hung every four hours. If available, use an infusion pump to regulate the number of drops per minute a patient receives.

stricted blood vessels? Starting nitroprusside in a patient with vasoconstriction will dilate his peripheral vessels. These vessels then accommodate the patient's blood volume, lowering his pressure. Excessive vasodilation without adequate volume replacement can lead to hypotension from hypovolemia.

Keep the I.V. solution wrapped in foil, because it's light-sensitive (see photo opposite). Stay at the bedside and check the patient's blood pressure every 5 minutes while the infusion is being started. If the situation permits, start an arterial pressure line, and regulate the flow of sodium nitroprusside to keep it at a certain level.

Nitroprusside is best run piggyback through a peripheral line with no other medication. It should be inserted at the injection site on the line closest to the patient. Do not regulate the rate of the main I.V. line while nitroprusside is running, because it will affect the infusion and you may inadvertently inject a bolus. Even small boluses of nitroprusside can cause a drastic drop in blood pressure. That's why running the drug through a CVP line is also unwise; when taking a CVP reading, you may infuse the nitroprusside faster than it was titrated to, again causing acute hypotension.

With all drugs like nitroprusside, that drastically lower blood pressure, you need emergency equipment on hand. If your hospital uses infusion pumps, these can best assure accurate infusion. If it doesn't have them, however, run the infusion through a mini-dripper. Check the rate every 15 minutes, once the patient becomes stable.

Suppose a hypotensive episode does develop: Immediately stop the I.V. infusion at the point closest to the patient, and notify the doctor. Nitroprusside usually wears off in 1-2 minutes. But lowering the patient's head and elevating his feet will help increase venous return and sometimes help restore normal pressure quicker. Usually, pressure returns on its own. However, the patient may need an increase in fluid volume, or — in some cases — an adrenergic stimulating drug. Take extra care to avoid a hypotensive episode in patients with coronary insufficiency or cerebral insufficiency. These conditions get worse with hypotension.

Patients on nitroprusside drips aren't usually ambulatory. However, if therapy continues for days, and the patient is ordered out of bed, be cautious. Ask him to dangle his legs first. If he feels dizzy, let him sit for several minutes before you

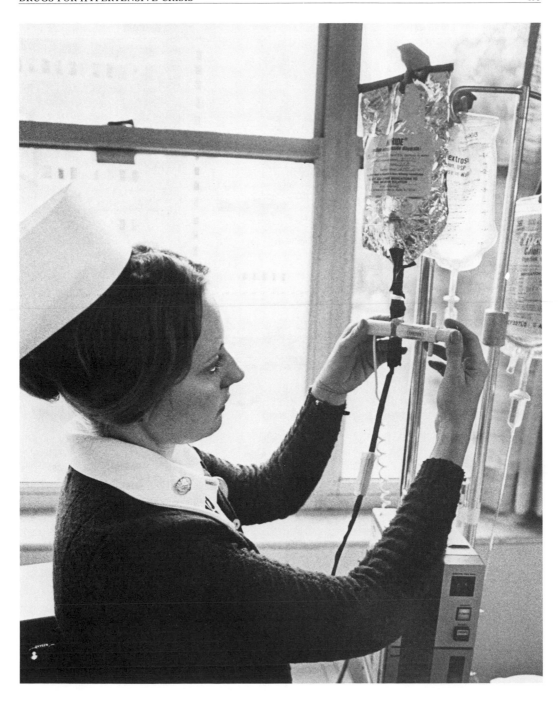

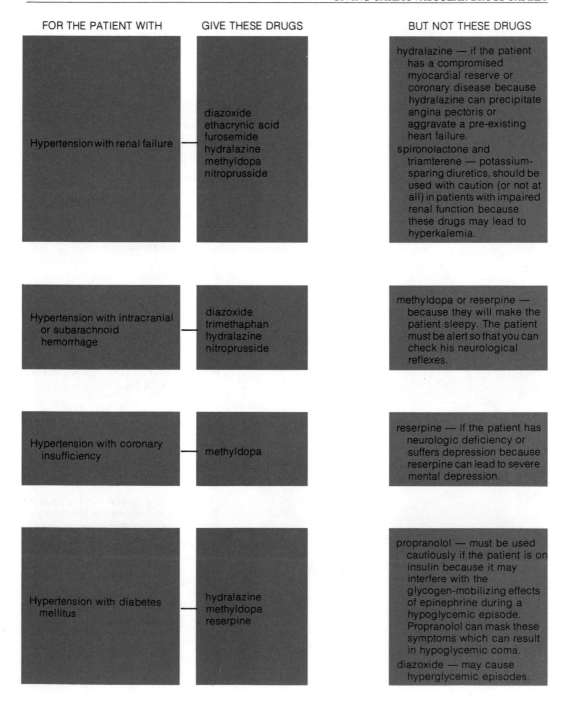

FOR THE PATIENT WITH	GIVE THESE DRUGS	BUT NOT THESE DRUGS
Hypertension with renal failure	diazoxide ethacrynic acid furosemide hydralazine methyldopa nitroprusside	hydralazine — if the patient has a compromised myocardial reserve or coronary disease because hydralazine can precipitate angina pectoris or aggravate a pre-existing heart failure. spironolactone and triamterene — potassium-sparing diuretics, should be used with caution (or not at all) in patients with impaired renal function because these drugs may lead to hyperkalemia.
Hypertension with intracranial or subarachnoid hemorrhage	diazoxide trimethaphan hydralazine nitroprusside	methyldopa or reserpine — because they will make the patient sleepy. The patient must be alert so that you can check his neurological reflexes.
Hypertension with coronary insufficiency	methyldopa	reserpine — if the patient has neurologic deficiency or suffers depression because reserpine can lead to severe mental depression.
Hypertension with diabetes mellitus	hydralazine methyldopa reserpine	propranolol — must be used cautiously if the patient is on insulin because it may interfere with the glycogen-mobilizing effects of epinephrine during a hypoglycemic episode. Propranolol can mask these symptoms which can result in hypoglycemic coma. diazoxide — may cause hyperglycemic episodes.

FOR THE PATIENT WITH	GIVE THESE DRUGS	BUT NOT THESE DRUGS
Malignant hypertension	diazoxide hydralazine nitroprusside reserpine trimethaphan	Any diuretic used alone or propranolol used alone — because in neither case are they effective. When used in conjunction with other antihypertensives, diuretics and propranolol are effective. Potassium-sparing diuretics, however, should be used cautiously or not at all.
Acute dissecting aneurysm of the aorta	nitroprusside reserpine trimethaphan	hydralazine — as it increases cardiac output.
Preeclampsia	diazoxide hydralazine methyldopa	methyldopa — can aggravate asthma, so check the patient's history before giving it. trimethaphan — should not be used because it can cross the placental barrier and endanger the fetus.
Acute left ventricular failure	diazoxide nitroprusside trimethaphan	hydralazine — because it increases ventricular workload.
Pheochromocytoma	phentolamine phenoxybenzamine propranolol	phentolamine — if the patient has myocardial infarction, a history of myocardial infarction, angina or coronary disease. Phentolamine has direct stimulant action on cardiac muscle and can cause tachycardia and cardiac arrhythmia with anginal pain. Phentolamine given I.V. can cause such extreme hypotension that the patient may risk myocardial infarction.

help him out of bed. Encourage him to change position slowly.

The nitroprusside ion gets converted to thiocyanate once it's in the bloodstream. So watch for signs of toxicity — nausea, anorexia, muscle spasms, fatigue, psychotic behavior, and confusion. If the drug is infused for longer than 72 hours, serum thiocyanate levels should be ordered every 72 hours. (Toxic thiocyanate levels are listed in Chapter 4.)

Initial adverse reactions to nitroprusside, besides excessive vasodilation and hypotension, are nausea, vomiting, sweating, restlessness, headache, palpitations, and substernal distress. Refer to the patient's baseline data when these occur, because some of these symptoms go with the hypertensive crisis itself. Close observation is needed to determine if symptoms like headache, nausea, and vomiting increase much with nitroprusside. If they do, notify the doctor.

Managing hypertension with renal failure
For severe hypertension secondary to acute or chronic glomerulonephritis, the following drugs are best: diazoxide, hydralazine, methyldopa, and nitroprusside.

If hydralazine is chosen, remember that it decreases blood pressure by directly dilating the vascular smooth muscles. It decreases diastolic blood pressure more than systolic. While it decreases blood pressure, it *increases* cardiac output and, so, the myocardial workload. Thus it's contraindicated in patients with coronary disease or compromised myocardial reserves, for it may precipitate congestive heart failure or coronary insufficiency.

While hydralazine decreases blood pressure, it doesn't concomitantly decrease renal blood flow. So it's excellent for renal insufficiency.

Hydralazine preferentially dilates arterioles rather than veins, minimizing the risk of postural hypotension.

Likely side effects to look for: headache, anorexia, nausea, dizziness, tachycardia, and moderate-to-severe palpitations. Hydralazine's myocardial effect can bring on anginal attacks and EKG changes that are characteristic of changes from myocardial infarction. They can usually be avoided if you slowly increase the dose. But if they do develop, notify a doctor and get a rhythm strip of an EKG. Usually, stopping the drug will end symptoms. But they shouldn't be forgotten, since slight impairment in myocardial function may have oc-

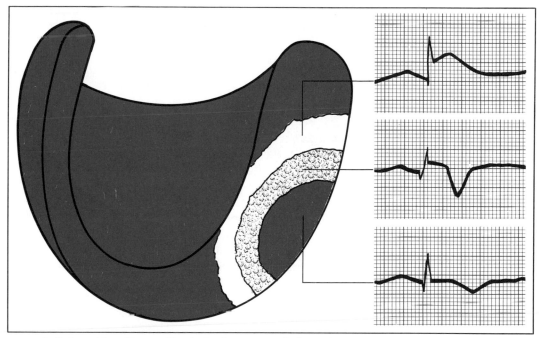

curred. Other side effects of hydralazine to watch for: edema, tremors, muscle cramps, and systemic lupus erythematosus.

Preeclampsia

A pregnant woman admitted for preeclampsia and elevated blood pressure is usually given one of these drugs: diazoxide, hydralazine, or methyldopa. If methyldopa is chosen, remember that it takes from 1-2 hours to start acting. Side effects include drowsiness and dryness in the mouth (which you can relieve with sour balls). Methyldopa can also aggravate asthma, so always take a thorough patient history before starting it. It can also produce orthostatic hypotension, so warn the patient not to change position suddenly. Keep her side rails up and the bed low. Show her the call buzzer so she can seek help before walking on her own. Because the patient on methyldopa can develop edema and weight gain from sodium retention, she may need diuretics. If she does, remember that diuretics increase the effects of methyldopa.

The metabolite of methyldopa excreted in the urine, may react with the oxidizing agents used to clean toilet bowls, producing a reddish color. This redness may be interpreted by

The heart of the matter
Myocardial infarction causes three changes in the wall of the heart; a zone of injury, indicated by an S-T segment elevation (Figure 1); a zone of ischemia, indicated by an inverted T wave (Figure 2); and a zone of tissue necrosis, indicated by a Q wave (Figure 3).

the patient as blood in her urine. Always tell her that this may occur if she continues on the drug after leaving the hospital.

Trimethaphan is not given during pregnancy. It can cause a meconium ileus in newborns.

Acute left ventricular failure

Here are the best drugs for this: nitroprusside, trimethaphan, and diazoxide. Hydralazine should be avoided because it only increases ventricular workload.

Diazoxide has a direct vasodilating effect. It increases cardiac output and rate, but because it lowers blood pressure, it doesn't increase myocardial work load. It can be given safely to patients with a decreased myocardial reserve. Because it also maintains renal blood flow, it works well in patients with renal insufficiency. It can cause sodium retention; so watch for signs of edema (especially in the legs) when the patient has been standing for long periods. Furosemide may be given to counteract such edema.

Another adverse effect of diazoxide is hyperglycemia. So, check urine glucose levels at least several times a day and notify a doctor of any changes. He may want to give insulin or another drug for the problem.

Though diazoxide promptly reduces blood pressure (usually within minutes), it doesn't permit gradual reduction. And precipitous reduction is particularly risky in coronary artery insufficiency or cerebral insufficiency.

Hypertension with intracranial or subarachnoid hemorrhage

The best drugs for this are diazoxide, trimethaphan, hydralazine, or nitroprusside, because none of them cause somnolence. Methyldopa and reserpine, on the other hand, cause somnolence. That, of course, would interfere with interpretation of neurologic signs, making it hard to tell if the patient's disorder was an infarct or hemorrhage. If it was an infarct, the decrease in blood pressure might aggravate the cerebral ischemia and worsen the neurologic deficit.

Malignant hypertension

For malignant hypertension, these drugs are best: diazoxide, nitroprusside, reserpine, or trimethaphan. Trimethaphan blocks both sympathetic and parasympathetic systems at the autonomic ganglia. Parasympathetic blocking can cause many

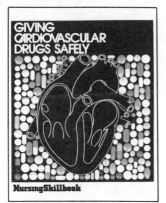
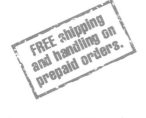
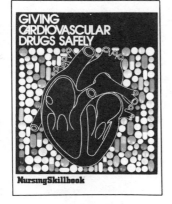
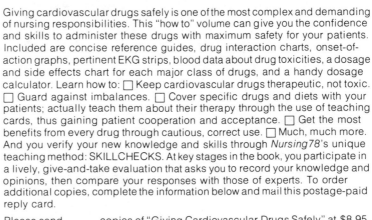

FIRST CLASS
PERMIT NO. 1903
HICKSVILLE, N.Y

BUSINESS REPLY MAIL

No Postage Stamp Necessary if Mailed in the United States

Postage will be paid by:

Nursing Skillbook

6 Commercial Street
Hicksville, N.Y. 11801

problems; for example, bladder atony, possibly necessitating catheterization. It may also cause bowel atony which may lead to a paralytic ileus, so pay special attention to bowel sounds and report changes to the doctor. This drug should not be given immediately postop, when bowel and bladder dysfunction are already present.

Because trimethaphan inactivates the pupillary reflexes, it may be difficult to do an accurate neurological check on the patient with intracranial hemorrhage or hypertensive encephalopathy. The effects of this drug are also orthostatic; elevating the head of the bed will enhance this.

Trimethaphan is contraindicated in patients with shock, severe arteriosclerosis, anemia, hypovolemia, polycythemia, kidney or liver damage, degenerative diseases of the central nervous system, severe cardiac disease, asphyxia, or any other condition in which there may be inadequate blood volume or circulation to a vital organ.

Because trimethaphan dilates the large veins, it can be used in patients with congestive heart failure.

Hypertension with coronary insufficiency

Methyldopa and reserpine are commonly used for this. They gradually decrease blood pressure, thus avoiding ischemia to the left ventricle. They also produce drowsiness, promoting rest, which further decreases left ventricular workload.

However, reserpine shouldn't be given to patients with neurologic deficits; it alters the level of consciousness and hampers clinical assessment. It's not given for depressed patients, who may be made more depressed by it (see Chapter 6). Large doses of reserpine can cause tachycardia, which may be misinterpreted as digitalis intoxication if the patient's also taking digitalis. Observe rate and rhythm of apical pulse. If the patient is in a monitoring unit, obtain rhythm strips every 8 hours.

Because of reserpine's sympatholytic effects, watch patients for signs of gastrointestinal bleeding. Reserpine can activate peptic ulcer. Another side effect is Parkinson-like symptoms, especially in the elderly. This usually stops when the drug is stopped.

Acute dissecting aneurysm of aorta

Reserpine, propranolol, trimethaphan are drugs of choice for this problem. As previously mentioned, trimethaphan can cause parasympathetic blocking.

Trimethaphan, propranolol, and nitroprusside may be used postoperatively, when blood pressures must be controlled to prevent rupture of newly sutured tissues. In this situation, the drugs are usually titrated to keep the patient slightly hypotensive. If you're titrating the drip to maintain low pressures, watch for signs of bleeding; a lower blood pressure may be due to hypovolemia caused by a blow-out of a graft or ruptured suture line. Usually, trimethaphan and nitroprusside are used for brief periods postoperatively and are titrated off soon after surgical repair.

Pheochromocytomas and MAO inhibitors

Patients with pheochromocytomas are usually treated with phentolamine. This drug blocks the vasoconstrictor effects of epinephrine. Given as an intravenous bolus or drip, it also demands constant attention by trained personnel. Observe the patient for signs of gastritis, because this drug can potentiate gastric bleeding.

Other adverse reactions to phentolamine include tachycardia, palpitations, and anginal pain.

A patient could also suffer a hypertensive crisis if he were on an MAO inhibitor drug and (1) ingested any sympathomimetic drug such as amphetamines, or (2) ate or drank foods that contained tyramine, for example, beer, Chianti wine, *pickled* herring, chocolate, chicken liver, yeast, coffee, or natural and aged cheeses.

Your role in a hypertensive crisis

No matter what the cause of hypertensive crisis, here's a standard procedure to follow. Take baseline vital signs soon after admission: blood pressure readings from both arms, apical pulse, respirations, and temperature. Also do a brief neurological examination: pupil checks for reaction to light and accommodation. Assess the patient's level of consciousness and orientation to time, person, and place. If he's experiencing a headache, try to place him in quiet surroundings away from loud noises and harsh lights. Help him into a comfortable position. Check his vascular status: Is he hydrated or dehydrated? As I said before, dilating a dehydrated patient can be disastrous unless you and the doctor are pre-

CLONIDINE
PATIENT TEACHING AID

Dear Patient:
Here's what you should know about the drug your doctor has prescribed for you.
Clonidine is used to treat high blood pressure. It will bring your blood pressure into a normal range and help keep it there.

To make sure you get the most from your therapy, follow these instructions carefully:

1. Take clonidine *only* as prescribed. Never skip a dose or change it in any way without an order from your doctor. *Never discontinue taking clonidine without specific instructions from your doctor. This is very dangerous.*

2. Stay on the diet your doctor has given you.

3. Tell *every* doctor who treats you that you are taking clonidine, especially if you will have surgery or will need an anesthetic for any reason.

4. Don't drink alcohol and don't take any other drugs, including nonprescription ones, without asking your doctor.

5. Clonidine may cause changes in your eyes. Have your eyes examined periodically by an ophthalmologist.

Call your doctor immediately if you notice any of the following: nervousness, muscle tremor, headache, nausea, increased salivation, constipation, dry mouth, drowsiness, dizziness, ankle swelling, weight gain, depression.

GUANETHIDINE
PATIENT TEACHING AID

Dear Patient:
Here's what you should know about the drug your doctor has prescribed for you.
Guanethidine is used to treat high blood pressure. It will bring your blood pressure into a normal range and help keep it there.

To make sure you get the most from your therapy, follow these instructions carefully:

1. Take guanethidine only as prescribed. Never skip a dose or increase, decrease, or change your dose in any way without an order from your doctor.

2. Stay on the diet your doctor has given you.

3. Tell *every* doctor who treats you that you are taking guanethidine, especially if you will have surgery or need an anesthetic for any reason.

4. Avoid sudden rising or prolonged standing. If you have been lying down or sitting for long periods of time, stand up slowly to avoid dizziness.

5. Avoid heavy exercise, and prolonged exposure to hot weather. Do not drink alcohol.

Call the doctor immediately if you notice any of the following: excessive diarrhea, impotence, nausea, muscle tremor, weight gain, ankle swelling, nasal stuffiness, dry mouth, or blurred vision.

pared and anticipate rapid hypotension.

Try to obtain a history from the patient or his family. Pay special attention to allergies, prior illnesses or conditions and anything that seems to precipitate the hypertensive crisis. Remember to be nonjudgmental and supportive of the family, especially if they were involved in an emotional incident with the patient.

During therapy, keep track of the patient's intake and output. Some drugs cause edema, interfere with renal blood flow, or cause urinary retention.

Patient education

Start teaching the patient and family as soon as possible. You can't do much in an ICU, but you start explaining the goal of therapy — lowering blood pressure. Stress that high pressure cannot be cured but controlled. Explain that control is a long-term goal, often requiring daily medication. Encourage the family and patient to talk about the crisis and how it may affect their future life style. Your own attitude toward the disease at this point can serve as a role model in developing the family and patient's attitudes and compliance for further treatment.

Simon Harris, the patient I told you about earlier, was switched from nitroprusside to a continuous infusion of the trimethaphan 1 gram/liter. His blood pressure then returned to normal, his neurological status improved to a state of slight right-sided weakness and normal level of consciousness, and he was eventually discharged on oral antihypertensives and diuretics.

When a patient is discharged on oral antihypertensives, you must teach him all he has to know about his drug — what precautions he must follow when taking it and what side effects may occur. Two of these drugs, guanethidine and clonidine, are described on patient teaching cards in this chapter. Two others, methyldopa and reserpine, are included in Chapter 6.

Thanks to powerful drugs — given cautiously but confidently by nurses and staff — patients like Mr. Harris can survive hypertensive crisis in just a few days. They can...if *you* do your job properly and notify the doctor when any of the problems I've discussed appear...and if you guard against a hypertensive crisis.

SKILLCHECK 4

1. Bertha Abbey, a 51-year-old horticulturist, has just returned to her room after having a benign breast cyst removed. Her stay in the recovery room was short and a check shows that she's responsive, her vital signs are normal, and her color is good. All seems well. Ten minutes later, however, you walk into her room and find that Mrs. Abbey is gasping and barely conscious. Her face is dusky. You immediately insure that she has an open airway, then you start checking her blood pressure. As you are doing this, Mrs. Abbey stops breathing and you find no palpable pulses. You start CPR and call a Code immediately. When the CPR team arrives, the doctor begins drug therapy. What drug is he likely to ask for first?

2. Leona Robards is a 56-year-old school teacher who was admitted to the CCU in hypertensive crisis. At the time of admission, her blood pressure was 210/130. To bring Mrs. Robards' blood pressure down to safe limits quickly, the doctor ordered I.V. nitroprusside to be run piggyback through a peripheral line. Mrs. Robards' blood pressure was checked every 5 minutes while the infusion was started; and after 1 hour, her blood pressure had dropped to 164/110. The other nurse in the room wants to check the patency of the main I.V. line and starts to open the main infusion clamp. Is there any reason she shouldn't?

3. Reginald Fitzwater is a 60-year-old novelist, who was rushed to the ER with a myocardial infarction. Shortly after being admitted to the CCU, where you are a nurse, he went into ventricular fibrillation. Basic life support measures were started and a Code was called. Mr. Fitzwater's ventricular fibrillation was converted to normal sinus rhythm by DC shock/400 w. sec. His blood pressure is palpable at 100 mm Hg and he is receiving I.V. dopamine. Now you notice a swelling above the insertion site. What do you do next?

4. You are a nurse in CCU where the doctor is working quickly to save 43-year-old Howard Rendell. Minutes earlier, he complained of severe chest pain and then suddenly went into ventricular standstill. Basic life support measures were begun and a Code was called.

The doctor has just given an I.V. injection of sodium bicarbonate, after which blood gases are drawn, and he is ready for the next emergency drug. Do you know what he will ask for?

5. Raymond Bertrand's blood pressure was 230/124 when he was brought to the emergency room by his son. Mr. Bertrand is a 60-year-old bartender with a long history of hypertension. The doctor immediately started him on nitroprusside I.V., then transferred Mr. Bertrand to the ICU, where his blood pressure began dropping steadily for three hours. However, the next time you check Mr. Bertrand's blood pressure it is 98/60. What do you do now?

6. When Oscar Connelly, a 66-year-old storekeeper, is brought into the emergency room, he is obviously very ill. His face is flushed, he seems confused, and he says his head is pounding. You take his blood pressure and find that it is 240/146. To bring Mr. Connelly's blood pressure down quickly, the doctor orders diazoxide I.V. *stat*. Moving briskly, you start an intravenous infusion of D5W and prepare the drug. How rapidly should diazoxide be injected?

7. You are a nurse on a CPR Code team and you are responding to a call from the medical/surgical floor. When you arrive, you find that Jonathan Winslow, a 72-year-old patient, has gone into ventricular standstill. Basic life support measures are already underway, but you notice that no I.V. is in place. Where would you start one and what size I.V. catheter would you use?

8. Agnes Bell, a 63-year-old housewife, is admitted to the hospital with a diagnosis of coronary insufficiency. During the night when you are checking her vital signs, you discover that her pulse rate is only 50/min. When you look at her chart, you find that her pulse rate has not been less than 56/min. on previous checks. Mrs. Bell now complains that she feels dizzy. Her blood pressure is only 96/60 and her apical pulse rate is 46/min. You call the doctor immediately. What emergency drug is he likely to order?

(Answers on page 168)

SKILLCHECK ANSWERS

ANSWERS TO SKILLCHECK 1 (Page 27)

1. b) 250-300 G, or from 9-11 ounces.
To convert to the metric system, remember that 1 ounce = 28.350 G

2. c) endocardium This smooth membrane lines the chambers of the heart and covers its valves and associated structures. It provides a smooth non-traumatic surface for the blood to pass over as it circulates through the heart.

3. a) tricuspid valve The mitral valve separates the left atrium from the left ventricle, and the pulmonic valve opens from the right ventricle to the pulmonary artery.

4. a) potassium Intracellular fluid is rich in potassium while extracellular fluid contains more sodium. When electrical current, generated by the heart's pacemaker, reaches the cell, it creates an ionic imbalance. Potassium moves out of the cell, while sodium migrates inward (depolarization).

5. c) sodium During depolarization, potassium moves out of the cell, while sodium migrates inward (see explanation in Answer 4).

6. b) 7 The presence of these glycogen-rich conduction pathways in the heart makes the conduction of electrical impulses more efficient.

7. a) AV node Impulses are delayed several milliseconds in the AV node to prevent the ventricles from being stimulated at inordinately rapid rates by the atria, and to permit adequate time for the ventricle to fill adequately before its systole.

8. b) 40-60 If the SA node fails, the AV node will take over pacemaker function in the heart, but at a slower rate. If the SA and AV nodes both fail, the ventricular muscles will continue to depolarize by themselves.

9. c) 1½-2 liters The arteriole's response to a vasodilating drug improves blood flow. The arteriole's response to a vasoconstricting drug decreases their capacity by 1-1½ liters and restricts blood flow.

10. b) the left circumflex artery The left anterior descending and the left circumflex artery arise from a common artery called the left main trunk.

11. a) right coronary artery This artery also supplies blood to the bundle of His and the inferior (diaphragmatic) wall of the left ventricle. In some people the left coronary artery is dominant.

12. a) adrenergic These responses can be mimicked or blocked by certain drugs. For example, the antiadrenergic drug, propranolol, blocks the response of beta receptors.

13. b) cholinergic When atropine or other anticholinergic drugs are given, the body's response to acetylcholine is blocked.

14. b) decrease the heart rate This can lead to bradycardia. However, the anticholinergic drug, atropine, can block overstimulation. It can increase the heart rate, which makes it useful as an antiarrhythmic.

15. b) constricting Cutaneous blood vessels have alpha receptors, unlike the skeletal muscle blood vessels that have beta 2 receptors. Skeletal muscle blood vessels respond to the release of norepinephrine by relaxing or dilating.

16. b) beta receptors That's why it's useful as an antiarrhythmic. However, it also constricts the bronchioles, so it's contraindicated for patients with asthma.

17. c) acetylcholine Atropine blocks the body's response to acetylcholine; for example, it increases the heart rate and constricts the blood vessels.

ANSWERS TO SKILLCHECK 2 (page 85)

Situation 1 — George Nicholson
Mr. Nicholson could develop digitalis toxicity for many reasons: (1) His hypothyroidism: This could increase or decrease his sensitivity to an average dose. (2) His age: Elderly patients usually show increased sensitivity to the drug. (3) Possible hypokalemia: When a patient takes a potassium-depleting diuretic without a potassium supplement, he may develop hypokalemia, increasing his chance of toxicity. Mr. Nicholson's cirrhosis probably won't affect his sensitivity to digitalis, because very little of the drug is metabolized in the liver.

Situation 2 — Albert Burke
Mr. Burke's symptoms suggest that he's hypersensitive to quinidine. When this happens, fever usually occurs from 3 to 20 days after the first dosage. Other allergic responses may accompany fever. Hypersensitivity to digoxin is uncommon.

Situation 3 — Francis Lloyd
Mr. Lloyd has dizziness and headache because he was digitalized too quickly for a person his age, weight, and heart rate. Furthermore, digoxin should be given orally — as any drug should — unless specifically ordered I.V. Always verify the route of administration when working with potent chronotropic drugs. If the patient is elderly and slender, his renal clearance may be impaired and, for him, small oral doses of digitalis are enough to control heart rate.

Situation 4 — Charity Wade
Mrs. Wade is doing what many patients do; trying to be her own doctor. Explain to her that she must take her prescribed drugs *exactly* as ordered and neither increase nor decrease the amounts without her doctor's knowledge. Tell her the diuretic is given to *prevent* and control the swelling of her ankles, as well as to help prevent fluid from building up in her lungs. Schedule her for another check-up soon, to both reinforce your teaching and check for edema.

Situation 5 — Pat Lafferty
Procainamide may increase the hypotensive effects of thiazide diuretics. Notify the doctor immediately and start checking Mr. Lafferty's blood pressure every ½ hour.

So Mr. Lafferty won't be frightened by the extra blood pressure checks, reassure him that they're helpful and probably will be continued only for a short time.

Situation 6 — James Spears
Mr. Spears' doctor will probably order an EKG and *stat* electrolytes. Because the patient is taking ethacrynic acid, one of the potassium-depleting diuretics, his skipped beats could be premature ventricular contractions from hypokalemia. If electrolyte values do show hypokalemia, the condition could be corrected with a potassium supplement. If the EKG shows PVCs, Mr. Spears may be transferred back to the CCU for continuous monitoring.

Situation 7 — Joe Alexander
Mr. Alexander is probably having an adverse reaction

to the lidocaine due to rapid I.V. infusion. Slow the drip immediately and call the doctor. Do not stop the infusion completely because this will increase Mr. Alexander's chances of developing more PVCs.

Are you also watching his EKG strips for changes in the PR interval? Lidocaine may prolong the conduction time from the SA node (sinoatrial). Report a change in PR interval if it increases above 0.20 seconds.

Situation 8 — Melvin Potter
Propranolol is probably causing Mr. Potter's difficulty. Because of the drug's beta blocking effect, the pulse doesn't increase with a drop in blood pressure. If propranolol is discontinued abruptly, it can increase the frequency and severity of anginal attacks and precipitate an MI. Dosage should always be reduced gradually. Monitor blood pressure, pulse, and respirations and lung sounds very closely when a patient is taking both propranolol and nitroprusside.

ANSWERS TO SKILLCHECK 3 (page 129)

Situation 1 — Maria Paone
First of all, if Mrs. Paone is pregnant, she shouldn't be taking reserpine, because it crosses the placental barrier and could damage the fetus. It is also secreted in breast milk. Tell the doctor immediately.

Secondly, Mrs. Paone's possible pregnancy — combined with her hypertension — could cause other complications: proteinuria, edema, excessive weight gain, and preeclampsia progressing to eclampsia.

Situation 2 — Rosie Salvatore
You can help Mrs. Salvatore by going over her diet and emphasizing the foods she *can* eat. Show her some of the excellent cookbooks containing low-fat recipes, and help her plan menus around the foods that will please her family. Be positive and encouraging, because patients like Mrs. Salvatore need a great deal of support. If you can, talk to her family about the problem. They may be able to reinforce your instructions.

Situation 3 — Lottie Gottwald
He will probably have Mrs. Gottwald checked for rheumatoid arthritis. But he may also suspect "hydralazine disease," which is a syndrome resembling arthritis that appears in some patient taking large doses of hydralazine over a prolonged period. This syndrome can progress to a lupus erythematosus-like ailment if the drug is not promptly discontinued.

Situation 4 — Peter VanZandt
Do a dip-stick test for blood in the urine. Notify Mr. VanZandt's doctor immediately if the test is positive for blood: The patient may be hemorrhaging. Also send a urine specimen to the lab for microscopic examina-

tion. Cloudy urine can be a sign of several conditions, including infection or inadequate fluid intake. Complete the assessment of Mr. VanZandt by checking for other signs of bleeding: nosebleeds, bleeding gums, petechiae or purpura, or bloody stools.

Situation 5 — Frank Rooney
Mr. Rooney's constipation and excess gas production may be caused by cholestyramine; these are just two of the side effects cholestyramine can produce. Tell the doctor. He may order a stool softener for Mr. Rooney and suggest that he increase his fluid intake.

Situation 6 — James LaBarr
Mr. LaBarr had orthostatic hypotension from the guanethidine. It's one of the drug's most common side effects, and usually most marked in the morning. Tell the doctor immediately, because he may want to reduce Mr. LaBarr's dosage. Explain to Mr. LaBarr that he can prevent dizziness by getting out of bed more slowly. Also warn him to avoid alcohol, heavy exercise, and prolonged exposure to hot weather. Because guanethidine also produces other side effects, ask Mr. LaBarr if he's had any other unusual symptoms, for example, diarrhea, nausea, fatigue, muscle tremor, nasal stuffiness, dry mouth, or blurred vision.

Situation 7 — Sara Henrich
Go directly to the doctor's original order — or call him — whenever you have a question about the drug a patient is getting. In this case, the original order read warfarin 25 mg P.O., *not* 2.5 mg P.O., as in the medication Kardex. Warfarin, like many other oral anticoagulants, has a larger initial dose than a maintenance dose; 25 mg should be Mrs. Henrich's first dose, and it's within the average first-dose range. Warfarin 2.5 mg would not give an adequate anticoagulant effect.

Situation 8 — Peter Lawler
With a gauze square, apply direct pressure to the cut on Mr. Lawler's chin and hold it firmly in place for several minutes. As you work to control the bleeding, remain calm and tell Mr. Lawler that it will soon stop. Reassure him that he will not bleed to death, a major fear of many patients who are taking anticoagulants. However, tell him that the clotting will take a little longer than usual.

When the bleeding has stopped, make a note of the incident on the chart and record the clotting time.

Situation 9 — Mabel Hegsted
First, find out exactly what the doctor has told her. Then copy or make up an appropriate patient teaching card on clonidine, using the sample in this Skillbook. Sit down with Mrs. Hegsted and discuss the information on it. For example, teach her to take clonidine only as prescribed and at the same time every day. Warn her

never to skip a dose or change it in any way without specific instructions from the doctor. See the patient teaching card on page 161 for the other important points to include in your teaching session. Ask Mrs. Hegsted's family to sit in on the discussion.

ANSWERS TO SKILLCHECK 4 (page 163)

Situation 1 — Bertha Abbey

The doctor will probably ask for an I.V. injection of sodium bicarbonate. It's the drug used to correct metabolic acidosis, which begins when a patient is in cardiac arrest. Acidosis must be treated promptly, because it depresses heart action and increases the risk of ventricular fibrillation. Also, the myocardium doesn't respond well to other CPR drugs or defibrillation when acidotic.

The initial sodium bicarbonate dose is 1 mEq/kg body weight. If the patient doesn't respond, the same dose is usually repeated in 10 minutes. Further doses are based on arterial blood gas and blood pH checks, which are necessary because too much sodium bicarbonate can cause alkalosis. Always keep an accurate record of the time and amount of each dosage.

Situation 2 — Leona Robards

Yes. You should never regulate the rate of the main I.V. line while nitroprusside is running, because it may affect the infusion and cause inadvertent injection of a bolus of nitroprusside. Even small boluses of this drug can lower a patient's blood pressure to a dangerous level. That's why running nitroprusside through a CVP line is also unwise. When taking a CVP reading you may infuse the nitroprusside faster than it was titrated to, causing acute hypotension. To check the patency of the main I.V. line, the nurse should have 1) checked the insertion site of the I.V. catheter for swelling or redness, 2) made sure the nitroprusside was infusing at the set rate. If there is no swelling or redness and the nitroprusside is infusing at the set rate, the I.V. is patent.

Situation 3 — Reginald Fitzwater

Discontinue the dopamine immediately and notify the doctor. The drug is probably infiltrating the subcutaneous tissue. When this happens, it may cause sloughing and necrosis. The doctor may order an injection of phentolamine to counteract the dopamine's adverse effects.

If the doctor wants you to continue giving dopamine to Mr. Fitzwater, start the new I.V. in a large vein, preferably in the antecubital fossa. Observe the injection site closely to prevent further subcutaneous drug infiltration.

Caution: Any time you must discontinue dopamine, monitor the patient's blood pressure closely, checking it every 5 minutes.

Situation 4 — Howard Rendell

The doctor will probably ask for intracardiac or intravenous epinephrine, a drug that makes the heart beat faster and contract more forcefully. Used with sodium bicarbonate and CPR, epinephrine can change a ventricular standstill to a rhythmic beat. It also increases blood pressure and blood flow to the brain. Take care never to let epinephrine come into direct contact with sodium bicarbonate, however, as this will inactivate the epinephrine.

Situation 5 — Raymond Bertrand

Stop the nitroprusside infusion immediately and call the doctor. Like all drugs that drastically lower blood pressure, nitroprusside can cause a hypotensive crisis. For this reason, you should always keep emergency equipment on hand when administering the drug. The patient may need an adrenergic stimulating drug or an increase in fluid volume to restore his blood pressure to normal.

Nitroprusside's effect usually wears off in 1-2 minutes, so when it's discontinued, the patient's blood pressure generally returns to a normal range without additional drug therapy. However, you can sometimes restore normal pressure quicker by lowering the patient's head and elevating his feet.

Situation 6 — Oscar Connelly

For best results, diazoxide should be injected intravenously within 10-20 seconds. For the first 5 minutes after the injection, check and record Mr. Connelly's blood pressure every minute. Then check and record it every 5 minutes, until it's stabilized. Report all your findings to the doctor. When he evaluates Mr. Connelly's condition, he may want you to give him another injection of diazoxide.

Situation 7 — Jonathan Winslow

Using D₅W, start the I.V. in a large vein, preferably one in the antecubital fossa. Use a large (16 gauge) catheter, because you will be injecting emergency drugs through it; a small gauge catheter could slip out of the vein wall. Tape the catheter securely in place, because life support measures may not permit the usual delicate handling of I.V. lines. If you are not able to start an I.V. immediately, the doctor will probably have to do a cutdown or insert a subclavian line.

Situation 8 — Agnes Bell

The doctor will probably order atropine I.V. *stat,* because it can increase blood pressure and cardiac output in patients with bradycardia and hypotension.

Always watch patients on atropine closely to determine the drug's effect on the heart rate. If it stays the same or decreases, the dosage may be too small (less than 0.3 mg) or the injection may have been given too slowly.

APPENDICES

THERAPEUTIC BLOOD LEVELS FOR CARDIAC DRUGS		
DRUG	APPROXIMATE THERAPEUTIC RANGE	
	Nanogram (1/1000 microgram)	Microgram
digoxin	1-2 nanogram/ml	
digitoxin	15-30 nanograms/ml	
lidocaine		2-5 micrograms/ml
phenytoin		6-18 micrograms/ml
procainamide		4-8 micrograms/ml
propranolol		0.05-0.15 micrograms/ml
quinidine		3-6 micrograms/ml

(Clinically toxic and subtherapeutic patients' levels sometimes overlap these ranges.)

Blood levels are excellent guides to therapy; however, patient observation for toxic symptoms, accurate medication administration, blood pressure and pulse monitoring remain essential to good patient care.

NURSES' GUIDE TO
PERIPHERAL VASODILATORS

GENERIC NAME	TRADE NAME	ROUTE AND DOSAGE	COMMON SIDE EFFECTS
tolazoline hydrochloride	Tolazoline Priscoline◇ Tolzol	P.O.: 25 mg 4-6 times daily, up to 50 mg 6 times daily (long-acting form: 80 mg q12h) S.C., I.V., I.M.: 10-50 mg q.i.d. Start with low doses and increase until optimum dose is reached (patient will flush)	Cardiac arrhythmias, anginal pain, hypotension, peptic ulcer exacerbation, GI disturbances, flushing, tingling, chills
cyclandelate	Cyclospasmol◇ Cyclandelate◇ Cyclanfor Cydel	P.O.: Initial dose 1200-1600 mg daily in divided doses with or before meals and at bedtime Maintenance 400-800 mg daily in 2-4 divided doses	GI distress, mild flushing, headache, weakness, tachycardia
isoxuprine hydrochloride	Isoxuprine Isolait Vasodilan Vasoprine	P.O.: 10-20 mg t.i.d. or q.i.d. I.M.: 5-10 mg b.i.d. or t.i.d.	Hypotension, GI disturbances, tachycardia, dizziness, palpitations
nylidrin hydrochloride	Nylidrin◇ Arlidin◇ Pervadil◇◇	P.O.: 3-12 mg t.i.d. or q.i.d.	Trembling, weakness, nervousness, nausea, vomiting, dizziness, palpitations
nicotinyl alcohol	Roniacol◇	P.O.: 50-100 mg t.i.d.; timed tablets — 150 mg a.m. and p.m.; elixir 5-10 ml t.i.d.	Transient flushing, gastric disturbances, minor skin rashes
niacin	Nicotinic acid◇ Niacin◇	P.O.: 100-500 mg daily in divided doses	Flushing, pruritus, GI distress, activation of peptic ulcers, jaundice, dry skin, hypotension, transient headache, tingling, dizziness, palpitations

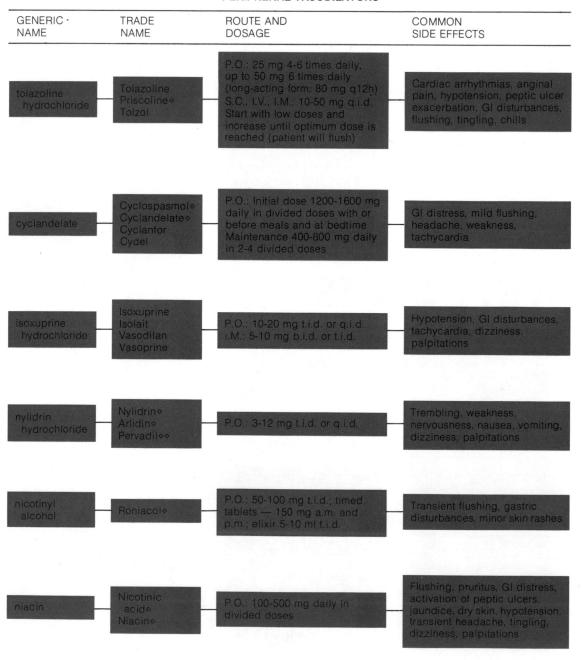

NURSES' GUIDE TO
PERIPHERAL VASODILATORS

GENERIC NAME	TRADE NAME	*ROUTE AND DOSAGE	COMMON SIDE EFFECTS
niacin (timed release)	Nicobid Diacin	P.O.: Nicobid — 125 mg a.m. and p.m. Diacin — 200 mg a.m. and p.m.	Flushing, GI distress, dry skin
papaverine hydrochloride	Papaverine◇	P.O., I.M., I.V.: 100-300 mg 3-5 times daily (I.V. preferred); 1-4 ml q3h (30 mg/ml), slowly over 1-2 min. in treatment of cardiac extrasystoles, 2 doses 10 min apart	GI disturbance, anorexia, increased perspiration, flushing of face, vertigo, headache, drowsiness, skin rash, intense facial flush, increased perspiration and depth of respiration, heart rate, slight rise in blood pressure, excessive sedation
papaverine hydrochloride (timed release)	Pavabid Cerebid Cerespan	P.O.: 150 mg q8-12h or 300 mg q12h	GI disturbance, vertigo, increased perspiration, headache, skin rash
ethaverine hydrochloride	Ethaquin Ethatab Cebral Eta-lent Isovex-100	P.O.: 100-200 mg t.i.d.	GI disturbance, dry throat, drowsiness, flushing, hypotension, headache, increased perspiration, respiratory depression, headache
ethaverine hydrochloride (timed release)	Circubid	P.O.: 150 mg b.i.d.	GI disturbance, dry throat, drowsiness, flushing, hypotension, headache, increased perspiration, respiratory depression, headache
dioxyline phosphate	Paveril phosphate	P.O.: 100-400 mg t.i.d. or q.i.d.	Mild nausea, flushing, increased perspiration, dizziness, abdominal cramping
ergot alkaloids, dihydrogenated	Hydergine◇ Deapril-ST	Sublingual: 1 mg t.i.d.	Sublingual irritation, transient gastric disturbances

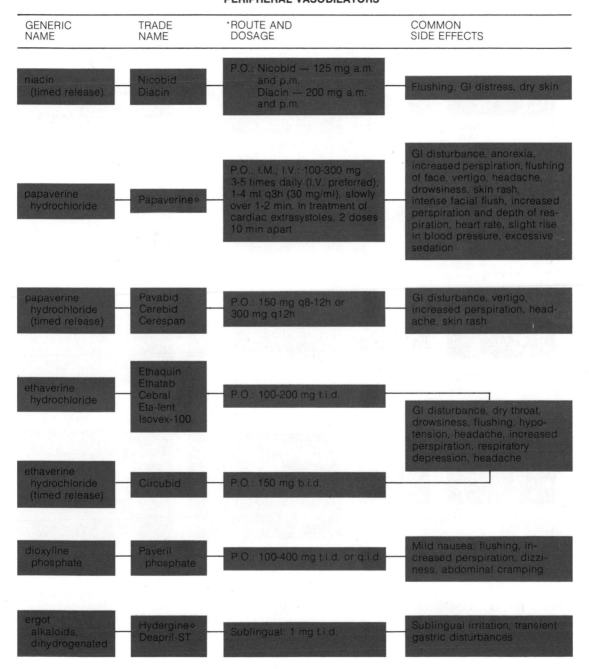

NURSES' GUIDE TO
COMMON ANTIHYPERTENSIVES

GENERIC NAME	TRADE NAME	ROUTE AND DOSAGE	COMMON SIDE EFFECTS
Miscellaneous			
phentolamine	Regitine	P.O.: 50 mg 4-6 times daily; I.V., I.M.: 5 mg 1-2h before surgery	Tachycardia, arrhythmia, and acute prolonged hypotensive episodes, weakness, dizziness, flushing, GI disturbance
phenoxybenzamine hydrochloride	Dibenzyline	P.O.: 20-60 mg daily (initially 10 mg daily, increased by 10 mg q4 days until desired effect obtained)	Nasal congestion, miosis, postural hypotension, tachycardia, inhibition of ejaculation, GI irritation
pargyline hydrochloride	Eutonyl◇	P.O.: 25-200 mg daily (in one dose)	Orthostatic hypotension, fluid retention, dry mouth, sweating, arthralgia, headache, insomnia, urinary difficulty, impotence, rash, muscle twitching, weight gain, GI disturbance
metoprolol tartrate	Betaloc◇◇ Lopresor◇◇	P.O.: 50-200 mg b.i.d. (initial dose is 50 mg b.i.d.; dose may be increased to 100 mg b.i.d. after the first week and by 100-mg increments every 2 weeks, not exceeding 200 mg b.i.d.)	Congestive heart failure, syncope, vertigo, postural hypotension, severe bradycardia, palpitations, chest pains, claudication, hot flashes, headache, insomnia, depression, GI disturbances, dyspnea, rash, pruritus, blurred vision

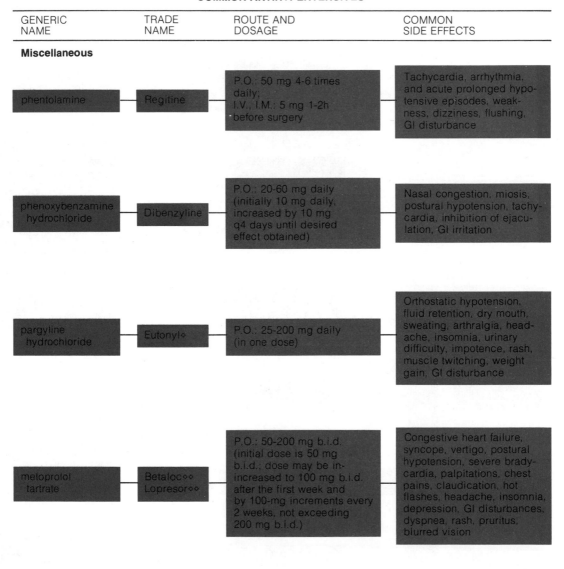

DOSAGE CALCULATIONS

I.V. FLOW RATE

---

1. Divide total 24-hour volume ordered by 3 to determine 8-hour amount to be infused.
2. Check I.V. set for drop factor (drops per cc).
3. Apply following formula.

$$\frac{\text{8-hour volume}}{100} \times \frac{\text{Drop Factor}}{5} + 1 = \text{Drops per minute}$$

Example: $\qquad \dfrac{1000 \text{ cc}}{100} \times \dfrac{15}{5} + 1 = 31 \text{ gtts./minute}$

CALCULATING ADULT DOSAGES

Liquid

$$\frac{\text{Desired Dosage}}{\text{Dose on hand}} \times \text{Quantity} = \text{Amount of solution to give}$$

Example: From a stock solution of 200 mg = 10 cc, how much solution is needed to give 75 mg of drug?

$$\frac{\text{Desired}}{\text{On Hand}} = \frac{75 \text{ mg}}{200 \text{ mg}} \times 10 \text{ cc} = 3.75 \text{ cc}$$

Tablets

$$\frac{\text{Desired dosage}}{\text{Dosage on hand}} = \text{Amount}$$

Example: Stock tablets of nitroglycerin are gr. 1/300. Desired dosage is gr. 1/150.

$$\frac{\text{Desire}}{\text{Have}} = \frac{1/150 \text{ gr.}}{1/300 \text{ gr.}} = \frac{1}{150} \times \frac{300}{1} = 2 \text{ tablets}$$

PATIENT TEACHING AID
YOUR FAT-CONTROLLED DIET — SHOPPING AND FOOD PREPARATION TIPS

If you're like most Americans, you probably eat too much of the wrong kind of fat; in other words, you eat fats that have more saturated components than unsaturated components.

Generally, foods that come from animal sources (for example, butter, whole milk, and meats) are high in saturated fats. Foods such as fish, poultry, nuts, and products containing *liquid* vegetable oil are higher in polyunsaturated fats.

Your doctor has given you a diet that is low in saturated fat. The foods listed on it are palatable and will fit into any family menu. To help you select and prepare these foods — as well as what to choose when eating out — we offer the following guidelines:

WHEN YOU SHOP:
- Meats.   Buy only lean cuts of meat. Eat less beef and add more fish and poultry to your diet. Veal cutlets, roasts, chops, and steaks are also good choices, if they are lean. If you want hamburger, select lean round steak and have the butcher grind it for you. Do not buy hamburger already ground, unless you are absolutely sure it is lean.

- Packaged and prepared foods. Always take the time to read the labels carefully before you buy. Sometimes, packaged or prepared foods contain eggs or saturated fats (for example, hydrogenated shortening) that should be avoided in your diet.

- Fruits and vegetables. These are good choices to include on your shopping list, as almost all fresh fruits and vegetables contain very little or no saturated fat.

- Breads and cereals. Buy enriched varieties of all breads, but read the labels carefully so you can aviod those that contain eggs, hydrogenated shortening, or whole milk. Be especially careful buying pastries, such as pie or coffee cake. These products almost always contain eggs and saturated fats. On the other hand, grain products such as rice or macaroni are usually low in saturated fats. However, read the label when you buy noodles; many varieties contain whole eggs.

- Dairy products. Almost all dairy products (whole milk, butter, cheese, ice cream, etc.) are high in saturated fat. However, you may buy skim milk, non-fat dry milk, and uncreamed cottage cheese. Avoid eggs, except in the quantities your doctor may allow. Look in the dairy case for commercial egg substitutes and use them whenever possible. Do not use butter or regular margarine. Use only margarines that are high in *liquid* oil.

- Desserts. Always read the label carefully when selecting packaged or prepared desserts. Avoid cakes, cookies, and dessert mixes that contain whole eggs, hydrogenated shortening, and whole milk. Angel food cake, which is made with egg whites, is a good alternative to other kinds of cake. Gelatin desserts and cornstarch puddings that you can make with skim or non-fat dry milk are also suitable. Take care selecting non-dairy coffee creamers, whipped toppings, or diet ice creams, because many of these products contain saturated fat. Read the label before you buy.

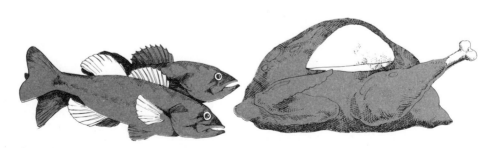

PATIENT TEACHING AID

YOUR FAT-CONTROLLED DIET — SHOPPING AND FOOD PREPARATION TIPS

WHEN YOU PREPARE FOODS:

- To adhere to your fat-controlled diet, you'll probably find it necessary to prepare most of your meals "from scratch," using low-fat recipes. Frozen entrees, TV dinners, packaged main dishes, baked foods, and dessert mixes contain more saturated fat than is allowed. Fortunately, many delicious recipes are available that will permit you to control the saturated fats in your diet. Look for low-fat cookbooks at your bookstore, or write to Standard Brands, Inc., 625 Madison Avenue, New York, New York 10022 for the booklet "Sensible Eating Can Be Delicious." Your doctor can order this book for you free. Otherwise, it is 50¢.

- Use only lean cuts of meat. Cut off all visible fat.

- When you use meat or poultry in a soup or stew, prepare the dish the day before use. Then chill it thoroughly and remove the fat that has hardened on the top before reheating.

- Broil meats, rather than fry them. If calories are not a problem, you may fry meat in a vegetable oil, such as corn oil.

- Brush meats, poultry, or fish with vegetable oil, rather than butter. Use the drippings as a sauce over the food when you serve it.

- Make cream sauces and gravies by using vegetable oil instead of butter; use skim milk or non-fat dry milk instead of whole milk or cream.

- Cook vegetables in a tightly covered pan, using a small amount of water. Do not add butter before serving, but use vegetable oil and herb seasonings for flavor.

- Substitute vegetable oil for shortening in recipes for muffins, pancakes, waffles, yeast breads, and pie crust. Substitute non-fat dry milk or skim milk when whole milk is needed.

- Make low-fat sherbet or ice milk using gelatin, non-fat dry milk and fruit juice. Low-fat ice cream substitutes are included in most low-fat cookbooks.

WHEN YOU EAT OUT:

- Staying on your fat-controlled diet can be difficult if you eat a lot of your meals away from home. Try to select a restaurant that offers a varied menu and let them know your needs.

- Choose these foods: fruit, fruit juice, clear soups, broiled or roasted meat, poultry or fish (without gravy or sauce); plain vegetables, salads (fruit or vegetable) without dressing, or with lemon juice; bread and rolls, skim milk, sherbet, gelatin, and angel food cake.

- Avoid these foods: butter, salad dressings, cream, sauces, gravy, cream soups, fatty meats, fried foods, casseroles, ice cream, pastries, and puddings.

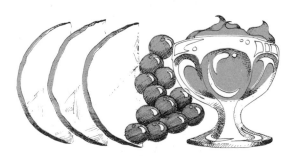

TABLE OF APPROXIMATE APOTHECARY/METRIC DOSE EQUIVALENTS

The Metric System is the official system of weights and measures of many hospitals. It is required that all medication orders be expressed in the Metric System. The following table is published as a convenience to nurses to assist in conversion of apothecary dosage expressions into the required metric expression.

LIQUID MEASURE

Apothecary	Approximate Metric Equivalent	Apothecary	Approximate Metric Equivalent
1 gallon	3,800 ml	4 Fl. ounces	120 ml
1 quart	950 ml	2 Fl. ounces	60 ml
1 pint	475 ml	1 Fl. ounce	30 ml
8 Fl. ounces (½ pint)	240 ml	15 minims	1 ml
		10 minims	0.6 ml

COMMON HOUSEHOLD MEASURES

1 teaspoon	5 ml	1 tablespoon	15 ml

WEIGHTS

Apothecary	Approximate Metric Equivalent	Apothecary	Approximate Metric Equivalent
1 ounce	30 G	1/6 grain	10 mg
15 grains	1 G	1/8 grain	8 mg
10 grains	600 mg	1/10 grain	6 mg
7½ grains	500 mg	1/12 grain	5 mg
5 grains	300 mg	1/20 grain	3 mg
1½ grains	100 mg	1/30 grain	2 mg
1 grain	60 mg	1/60 grain	1 mg
¾ grain	50 mg	1/100 grain	600 mcg
½ grain	30 mg	1/150 grain	400 mcg
⅜ grain	25 mg	1/200 grain	300 mcg
¼ grain	15 mg	1/250 grain	250 mcg
		1/300 grain	200 mcg

For scientific use or precise calculating, the following exact metric weights and measures are used:

Liquid Measure			Weight		
1 Fl. ounce	=	29.57 ml	1 Kilogram	=	2.2 pounds
1 pint	=	473.167 ml	1 ounce	=	28.35 G
1 milliliter	=	16.23 minims	1 G	=	15.432 grains
			1 grain	=	64.8 mg

Courtesy: Temple University Hospital, Philadelphia, Pa.

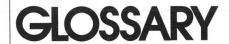

GLOSSARY

acidosis, metabolic — a condition in which there is an excess of hydrogen ions in the blood, due to loss of base or retention of non-carbonic acids

adrenergic — a term used to describe the fibers which release and the receptors which respond to catecholamines.

aneurysm — a sac formed when blood dilates the walls of an artery or vein.
Acute dissecting: a steady accumulation of blood escaping into the intimal layers of an artery.

angina pectoris — chest pain due to heart muscle receiving insufficient supply of oxygen.

antiadrenergic — blocking adrenergic response (see adrenergic).

antilipemics — drugs used for the reduction of fats or lipids in blood.

arrhythmia — any disturbance in the rate, rhythm, or conduction of the heart.

asystole — ventricular standstill.

atherosclerosis — narrowing of the lumen of arterial walls. The accumulation of fatty plaques.

atony — lack of normal muscle tone; i.e., bowel or bladder.

autonomic nervous system — that part of the nervous system that governs involuntary muscular action.

azotemia — increased concentrations of nitrogenous products in the blood, especially urea.

bigeminal rhythm — beats which occur in pairs — one normal, one premature (atrial or ventricular). Related to regularly occurring premature contractions.

bradycardia — abnormal slowness of heart rate with fewer than 60 beats per minute.

cardioversion — restoration of rapid, abnormal rates and/or rhythms to normal sinus rhythm by drug or electrical countershock.

catecholamines — group of neurohormones produced largely by the adrenal medulla and adrenergic nerve endings having an adrenergic effect on autonomic nervous system.

cholinergic — a term used to describe the fibers which release and the receptors which respond to acetylcholine.

chronotropic — stimulation of the heart affecting the time or rate of contractions.

conduction — transmission of electrical impulses through special conduction fibers in the heart causing heart muscle contraction.

contractility — tightening or shortening of muscle fibers in response to suitable stimulus.

Coombs' tests — laboratory tests to 1) determine certain antibody-antigen reactions; 2) differentiate between certain hemolytic anemias; 3) determine certain blood types, including Rh factor; and 4) to help diagnose erythroblastosis fetalis.

diabetogenic — producing diabetes.

diaphoretic — promoting excessive perspiration.

diastole — the phase of the heart cycle when it relaxes and fills with blood.

electrophoresis — a laboratory method used to analyze the plasma's protein content.

encephalopathy — abnormal brain function without underlying abnormality.

enteric mucosa — mucous membrane lining intestinal tract.

enterohepatic circulation — the process in which bile salts or drugs are absorbed from the intestine and excreted by the liver.

fascicle — a bundle of nerve or muscle fibers such as the left and right bundle branches in the ventricles.

fibrillation — abnormal, rapid, chaotic arrhythmia of either atria or ventricles which prevents efficient myocardial contractility.

ganglion — a knot-like mass of nerve cell bodies located outside the central nervous system.

glomerulonephritis — inflammation of the capillaries in the glomeruli of the kidney.

half-life — the length of time it takes for an amount of drug in the blood to be reduced by half.

heart block, first degree — a condition occurring when electrical energy impulses are delayed at the AV node, disrupting normal conduction. Prolonged P-R interval on EKG.

hemiparesis — paralysis affecting one side of the body.

hypercholesteremia — excess of cholesterol in the blood.

hyperkalemia — excessive potassium in the blood.

hyperlipidemia — abnormally high levels of lipids (fats) in the blood.

hyperlipoproteinemia — excess of lipoproteins in the blood.

hypertensive crisis — an elevated blood pressure of 200/120 or greater.

hypoglycemia — below normal blood sugar.

hypokalemia — abnormally low levels of potassium in the blood.

IHSS — (idiopathic hypertrophic subaortic stenosis) a congenital heart defect characterized by hypertrophy of the left ventricular outflow tract and a thickening of the muscle of the left ventricle and ventricular septum.

inotropic — affecting force or energy of cardiac contraction.

irritability — ability of the heart muscle to respond to stimuli.

myocardial infarction — tissue necrosis caused when an area of the heart has its blood supply cut off.

myocardial ischemia — a condition resulting from blood and oxygen starvation of the heart muscle.

orthopnea — inability to breathe except in an upright position.

orthostatic hypotension — Rapid lowering of blood pressure when position is changed from supine to standing.

palpitations — awareness of excessively rapid heartbeats.

parasympathomimetic — produces effect resembling stimulation of parasympathetic nerve fibers.

paroxysmal atrial tachycardia — (PAT) an arrhythmia characterized by the sudden onset of rapid, regular heartbeats in excess of 150-250 beats per minute.

peripheral vascular resistance — depends on size of vessel and viscosity of fluid in measuring force of blood flow.

pheochromocytoma — a tumor of the adrenal medulla that, by overproducing adrenal hormones, causes hypertension.

PR interval — on an EKG, this indicates atrioventricular conduction time. The interval is measured from the onset of the P wave to the beginning of the QRS complex.

preeclampsia — toxic condition of late pregnancy characterized by edema, albuminuria and hypertension.

premature atrial contraction — (PAC) an atrial contraction which occurs too early in the cycle and arises from irritable or ectopic pacemaker activity in the atria.

prothrombin — a glycoprotein that's converted to thrombin in the second stage of blood coagulation.

presso-receptors — nerve endings located in the aortic arch and the carotid sinuses that are sensitive to changes in blood pressure and react by slowing or speeding up rate of cardiac contractions.

pyelonephritis — inflammation of the kidney and its pelvis.

QRS complex — on an EKG, this segment reflects ventricular depolarization.

QT interval — on an EKG, this represents the time (in the cardiac cycle) required for ventricular depolarization and repolarization.

refractory — resistant to treatment.

systole — the contraction phase of the heart muscle that forces blood from the ventricles into the pulmonary artery and aorta.

tachycardia — heart rate greater than 100 beats per minute. It may be sinus, atrial, junctional or ventricular in origin.

tachycardia, reflex — an impulse (triggered elsewhere in the body) that directly affects the heart causing it to beat rapidly.

trigeminal rhythm — occurs in threes, as two normal beats followed by one premature beat.

triglyceride — in the bloodstream, a glycerol to which fatty acids are attached.

vasodilator — an agent that relaxes (dilates) venous or arterial vessel walls.

vasopressor — an agent that stimulates generalized vaso-constriction, usually increasing blood flow to the body's vital organs.

INDEX

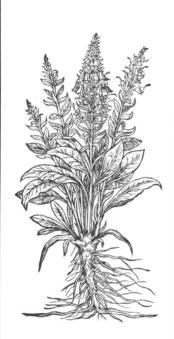

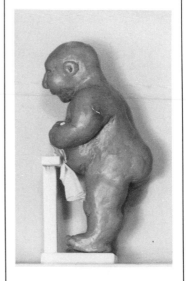

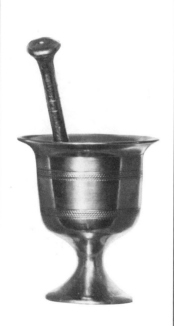

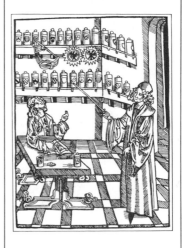

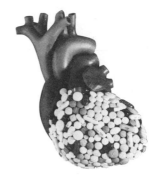